The Diabetic Diary 2003

The Diabetic Diary 2003

L. D. Sutton, M.D., Ph.D.

Writers Club Press

New York Lincoln Shanghai

The Diabetic Diary 2003

Writers Club Press
an imprint of iUniverse, Inc.

For information address:
iUniverse
2021 Pine Lake Road, Suite 100
Lincoln, NE 68512
www.iuniverse.com

ISBN: 0-595-25634-1

Printed in the United States of America

CONTENTS

LIST OF ABBREVIATIONS

ALT ....Alanine aminotransferase

AST ....Aspartate aminotransferase

BMI ....Body mass index

BUN ....Blood urea nitrogen

CK..Creatine Kinase

CRT..Creatinine

dL ....deciliter

HDL-C..High density lipoprotein cholesterol

Hg..Mercury

hr ....Hour

in ....Inches

K..Potassium

Kg..Kilograms

lb..Pounds

LDL-C..Low density lipoprotein cholesterol

m ....Meters

mg ....Milligrams

min ....Minute

mm ....Millimeters

Trig..Triglycerides

μg ....Micrograms

INTRODUCTION

Diabetes continues to rise in America. It is now estimated that 7.3 % of our population is afflicted. That is 21 million people! CDC projections estimate that by the year 2010 the incidence will be 10% or 30 million people. This is clearly a national epidemic of an unprecedented scale.

Yet studies continue to show that diabetics are not receiving adequate care and education. Scientific clinical studies continue and have provided the foundations for a well-defined, but rather complex regimen for health maintenance management of diabetics. *The Diabetic Diary 2003* simplifies this regimen and is the means by which the diabetic patient can take control of his/her own medical management.

Myths about diabetes abound. I frequently meet diabetic patients who tell me their doctor has told them they must avoid carbohydrates and sugar. This is patently wrong! A diet wherein less than 50 to 60% of calories are derived from carbohydrates is a diet that enhances diabetic complications and mortality. And sugar should be counted just the same as any other carbohydrate. See the dietary section on page 19.

Very frequently I meet type 2 diabetic patients who do not check their blood sugars often, if at all. This is poor diabetic management. Last year a study was conducted that concluded that the majority of time when physicians accuse their patients of noncompliance with their diets or medications, it is in fact poor medical management by the physician. This makes perfect sense given that many type 2 diabetics aren't measuring their home blood sugars and recording them. How then can the doctor (or the patient) know if the prescribed medications are working properly?

There is not a lot of reading in this book, but what is here is important. The text concisely and simply summarizes general treatment goals for the diabetic patient. Read the text and review it often. Knowing the information in this book will keep you well ahead of the pack with respect to diabetic management.

Most importantly, fill out the tables in this book. Diabetic management requires diligence. Check your blood sugars often and record them. Get your laboratory testing done on schedule and record the results. Get your examinations done and record them. If you do this, you and your doctor will be able to readily determine if you're meeting your health maintenance goals.

This book is not intended to prescribe treatment. Because treatment must be individualized, you should consult with your physician for recommendations concerning your treatment requirements.

Thank you for choosing THE DIABETIC DIARY 2003. It is an honor to be chosen to participate in your health care delivery.

PERSONAL INFORMATION

► Fill in the information as directed.

► **Take this book with you for all physician and emergency room visits.** The information in this section, and the Past Medical History and Medications sections provide important and sometimes critical information to health care providers concerning your medical management. The information as presented in this book is designed to be as efficient as possible for your physicians.

► Diabetes that was formerly referred to as Juvenile, Type I or Insulin Dependent is now correctly referred to as **Type 1.**

► Diabetes that was formerly referred to as Adult, Type II or Noninsulin Dependent is now correctly referred to as **Type 2.**

► There are other types under special medical circumstances. If your disease is not Type 1 or Type 2, then fill in your specific diagnosis.

Name _____

Date of birth _____

Date first diagnosed with diabetes _____

Type 1 or 2 diabetes? (circle one) or List other type: _____

List **allergies** to medicines:_____

_____

_____

_____

Do you use **insulin** to control your diabetes? YES or NO

Current address: _____

_____

_____

_____

EMERGENCY NOTIFICATION:

Name _____

Address _____

_____

_____

Telephone number _____

PERSONAL PHYSICIAN: Name _____

Telephone number _____

MEDICAL AND SURGICAL HISTORY

▶ Fill in the information as directed. Just check mark the diseases that you have or have had. Leave the rest of the spaces blank. This will allow you to check mark additional diagnosis as they occur.

▶ While this section is designed to give your doctor the past medical history pertinent to your health care, space is left at the end of this section for additional history. You may also use this section to elaborate on the diagnosis you check. For example you may list the number and dates of each heart attack or your bypass operation or your stroke(s).

▶ Please keep this section as legible as possible. Clutter may lead to misinterpretation and compromise your medical outcome.

MEDICAL HISTORY

Tobacco: Currently smoke _____ packs of cigarettes per day.

Quit smoking in the year _____

I use other tobacco products. _____

I have never used tobacco products _____

I have _____ **alcoholic** drinks per DAY / WEEK / OCCASIONAL.

Check all diagnosis that apply:

Stroke (Brain attack) ...._____

Transient ischemic attacks (TIA, mini-strokes) ...._____

Stroke (Cerebral Hemorrhage) ...._____

Seizures (epilepsy) ...._____

Coronary artery disease(Heart disease) ...._____

Previous heart attacks ...._____

Angina ...._____

Congestive heart failure.._____

Heart valve disease ...._____

Mitral valve prolapse ...._____

High blood pressure ...._____

Arrhythmia (irregular heart beat) ...._____

Peripheral vascular disease (claudication)..........................._____

Deep venous thrombosis (DVT)..._____

Cataracts..._____

Diabetic retinopathy ...._____

Macular degeneration ...._____

Legally blind ...._____

Asthma ...._____

COPD (Emphysema) ...._____

Diabetic gastroparesis ...._____

Heart burn (GERD) ...._____

Hiatal hernia ...._____

Peptic ulcer disease ...._____

Gastrointestinal (GI) bleeding..................................._____

Diverticulitis ...._____

Irritable bowel syndrome..._____

Hernia ...._____

Kidney disease.._____

Diabetic foot disease ...._____

Number of pregnancies ...._____

Number of deliveries..._____

Number of miscarriages ...._____

Diabetic neuropathy ...._____

Obesity ...._____

Osteoarthritis ...._____

Rheumatoid arthritis..._____

Lupus erythmatosis ...._____

Osteoporosis .... _____

Hypothyroidism .... _____

Hyperparathyroidism .... _____

Addison's disease .... _____

Liver failure.. _____

Gall stones (cholelithiasis) .... _____

Gall bladder inflammation (cholecystitis) .... _____

Compression fractures... _____

Cancers:

      Brain tumor .... _____

      Breast .... _____

      Lung .... _____

      Colon .... _____

      Prostate .... _____

      Cervical.. _____

      Uterine .... _____

      Ovarian.. _____

      Testicular .... _____

      Kidney .... _____

      Bladder .... _____

      Liver .... _____

      Pancreas .... _____

Thyroid..._____

Multiple endocrine neoplasia ...._____

Leukemia ...._____

Lymphoma ...._____

Skin, melanoma ...._____

Skin, basal cell.._____

Skin, squamous cell....................................._____

Infectious disease:
HIV positive ...._____

AIDS ...._____

Hepatitis A ...._____

Hepatitis B ...._____

Hepatitis C ...._____

Hepatitis, non-A, non-B, non-C ...._____

Rheumatic fever ...._____

Additions, clarifications and hospitalizations:

_____

_____

_____

_____

_____

_____

SURGICAL HISTORY

Check all procedures that apply:

Appendectomy ...._____

Gall bladder (cholecystectomy) ...._____

Cataract repair ...._____

Colonoscopy.._____

Upper endoscopy (EGD) ...._____

Tonsillectomy ...._____

Adenoidectomy.._____

Cesarean section ...._____

Coronary artery bypass graft (CABG, Heart bypass) ...._____

Cardiac catheterization (angiography) ...._____

Coronary artery angioplasty (balloon) ...._____

Coronary artery stent placement ...._____

Bone marrow biopsy ...._____

Breast biopsy.._____

Breast lumpectomy ...._____

Mastectomy ...._____

Transurethral retrograde prostatectomy (TURP) ...._____

Prostatectomy ...._____

Bone marrow biopsy ...._____

Liver transplant.._____

Heart transplant ...._____

Kidney transplant ...._____

Pancreas transplant ...._____

Bone marrow transplant ...._____

Bone transplant (autologous) ...._____

Skin graft ...._____

Sinus surgery..._____

Lung tumor removal ...._____

Lung lobectomy ...._____

Brain tumor removed ...._____

Femoral-popliteal bypass graft.._____

Splenectomy ...._____

Dental extraction ...._____

List other operations and surgical procedures:

_____

_____

_____

_____

_____

_____

_____

CURRENT MEDICATIONS

▶ List the names of your medications, dosage and times of day taken. If you take different doses of the same medication at different times, feel free to list these on separate lines. Again, legibility counts.

▶ In the insulin section fill in only those that apply and leave the rest blank. For specialized regimens, sliding scale regimens and insulin pump settings be as exact and legible as possible; giving type of insulin and when administered.

▶ Generally a diabetic should be on medications to control blood sugar, a daily aspirin, lipid controlling medications and possibly blood pressure medications with special preference towards medications called angiotensin converting enzyme (ACE) inhibitors for renal (kidney) protection. Check with your physician.

CURRENT MEDICATIONS

Name of Medicine	Dosage	Taken Times Daily
_____	_____	_____
_____	_____	_____
_____	_____	_____
_____	_____	_____
_____	_____	_____
_____	_____	_____
_____	_____	_____
_____	_____	_____
_____	_____	_____
_____	_____	_____
_____	_____	_____
_____	_____	_____
_____	_____	_____

Name of **INSULIN** used: _____

Regular	Morning units _____	Evening units _____
NPH (lente)	Morning units _____	Evening units _____
Ultra Lente	Morning units _____	Evening units _____
70/30	Morning units _____	Evening units _____

Insulin pump settings: _____

_____

_____

_____

Sliding scale and specialized regimens: _____

_____

_____

_____

_____

_____

_____

_____

_____

_____

_____

_____

_____

_____

_____

IMMUNIZATIONS

▶ Enter the dates for your most recent vaccination(s).

▶ Diabetics are considered to have impaired immune function. Therefore, they may have worse cases of infectious diseases, making them sicker and increasing likelihood of death. Immunizations play an important role in diabetic management.

▶ At a minimum diabetics should have:
  1) An annual influenza vaccination.
  2) One lifetime pneumococcus vaccination.
  3) Current tetanus vaccination.

INFLUENZA

▶ Vaccinate annually. Each year 20 million Americans catch the flu and 20,000 of them die!

▶ All diabetic patients should receive an annual influenza vaccine beginning each September. Contra-indications include allergy to egg products or other components of the influenza vaccine and Guillain-Barré syndrome within 6 weeks of a previous influenza vaccination. The vaccination cannot cause influenza or other respiratory diseases. The most common side effect is soreness at the injection site.

▶ Prophylaxis with anti-influenza drugs such as Symmetrel (amantadine) and Flumadine (rimantadine) may be used if allergy prevents immunization. These drugs are effective only against Influenza A. Tamiflu (oseltamivir) is approved for prophylaxic use. To date Relenza (zanamivir) is only approved for treatment of influenza infections, but presumably would be effective as an influenza prophylactic. Tamiflu and Relenza are effective against both Influenza A & B.

▶ *Influenza vaccination does not guarantee that one will not catch the flu!*

1. The trivalent vaccine is constituted of strains of Influenza A & B most likely to circulate in the USA during influenza season. Exposure to another strain of influenza might result in infection.

2. A vaccinated patient may become infected with a strain immunized against, but the disease should not be as severe.

3. Many other viruses cause influenza-like symptoms, but are generally referred to as "the flu."

Influenza vaccination date _____/_____/_____

PNEUMOCOCCUS

▶ A.K.A. Streptococcus pneumoniae. One time vaccination.

▶ All diabetics should receive at least one pneumococcal vaccination. Indications for repeat vaccination include:

1. Patients over the age of 65 that were less than 65 years old at the time of their initial vaccination *and* more than 5 years have elapsed since their initial vaccination.

2. Other indications for repeat vaccination may include nephrotic syndrome, chronic renal disease and immunocompromised states.

▶ Up to half of patients receiving pneumococcal vaccination experience soreness at the injection site. Severe reactions are rare.

▶ It is well established that the pneumococcal vaccine is effective in reducing life threatening disease due to pneumococcal blood infection (pneumococcal bacteremia). Its effectiveness in preventing other pneumococcal disease remains uncertain, including pneumococcal pneumonia. One should also remember that other bacteria and viruses can cause pneumonia. *It is therefore a misnomer to refer to this vaccination as the "pneumonia shot."*

Pneumococcal vaccination date(s): #1 _____/_____/_____

#2 _____/_____/_____

TETANUS

▶ Boost every 10 years. Complete series may be indicated.

▶ Diphtheria-tetanus toxoid should be administered every 10 years. If over 30 years have elapsed or if one has never been immunized, the whole series should be administered. Contra-indications to tetanus vaccination include allergy to any component of the vaccine.

Tetanus vaccination date: #1 _____/_____/_____

#2 _____/_____/_____

#3 _____/_____/_____

DIETARY RECOMMENDATIONS
MEDICAL NUTRITION THERAPY

▶ Dietary recommendations have changed dramatically during the past century resulting in much confusion amongst physicians. The following is what the American Diabetic Association currently recommends.

▶ **Calorie Reduction:** A modest calorie reduction of 250 to 500 Calories daily below calculated maintenance requirements. A weight loss of 10 to 20 pounds is generally recommended regardless of starting weight. Check with your physician or dietician.

▶ **Protein:** 10 to 20% of your calories should come from dietary protein. Certain diseases such as renal failure may reduce the recommended intake. Check with your physician.

▶ **Fat:** Less than 30% of your calories should come from fat.
Saturated fat: <10%. For cholesterol reduction <7%.
Polyunsaturated fat: <10%
Monounsaturated fat: 10-15%

▶ **Cholesterol:** <300 mg/day. For cholesterol reduction < 200 mg/day.

▶ **Carbohydrates:** Obtain the remainder of your calories from this food group.
Sugar (sucrose): Sugar should be treated gram for gram like any other carbohydrate. *Diabetics can have their cake and eat it, too!*
Fructose: Fructose, especially naturally occurring is acceptable, as is its use in modest quantities for sweetening. However, large quantities should be avoided as it has been shown to increase LDL (bad) cholesterol.

▶ **Fiber:** 20-35 grams of combined soluble and insoluble fiber daily.

▶ **Sodium:** Recommendations vary between ≤2,400 mg and 3,000-mg daily consumption. If you have hypertension it is recommended that your intake be decreased to ≤2,000-mg daily.

▶ **Complications:** Underlying medical conditions may require your doctor to prescribe diets that vary from the above.

HOME BLOOD SUGAR MONITORING RECORDS

▶ Enter the times blood sugars were tested and the corresponding values.

▶ All home glucometers measure blood sugar from whole blood. However, some have been calibrated to give plasma values which run a little higher when compared to whole blood. It is therefore important for you to know which type of glucometer you have. Use the appropriate section for your glucometer to interpret your readings.

▶ Goal values (approximate) **whole blood values:**

1. **Fasting =100 ± 20 mg/dL.** Usually first morning. No food or drink for ≥ 8 hours.

2. **Before meals = 100 ± 20 mg/dL.** Essentially the same as fasting.

3. **Bedtime = 120 ± 20 mg/dL.**

4. **After meals = 140 mg/dL.** Two hours after meals. I found no data specifically addressing changes in this value.

▶ Goal values (approximate) **plasma values:**

1. **Fasting =110 ± 20 mg/dL.** Usually first morning. No food or drink for ≥ 8 hours.

2. **Before meals = 110 ± 20 mg/dL.** Essentially the same as fasting.

3. **Bedtime = 130 ± 20 mg/dL.**

4. **After meal = 150 mg/dL.** Two hours after meals. I found no data specifically addressing changes in this value.

▶ **Type 2 diabetics** should check their blood sugars daily if they are using insulin or sulfonurea medications (such as Amaryl, Glucotrol, Micronase, DiaBeta, Orinase, Tolinase or Diabinese). Measurements should be sufficiently frequent to optimally achieve glucose goals. Data have shown more frequent monitoring results in significantly lowered glycosylated hemoglobin levels. Type 2 diabetes is a progressive disease requiring frequent medication changes. My personal opinion is daily fasting and bedtime checks, at a minimum.

▶ **Type 1 diabetics** should check their sugars as prescribed by your physician to fit your insulin regimen. Generally, Type 1 diabetics should measure their blood sugars 3 or 4 times daily.

HOME BLOOD SUGAR MONITORING RECORDS

JANUARY

► Goal values (approximate) <u>**whole blood values:**</u>
1. **Fasting =100 ± 20 mg/dL.** Usually first morning. No food or drink for ≥ 8 hours.
2. **Before meals = 100 ± 20 mg/dL.** Essentially the same as fasting.
3. **Bedtime = 120 ± 20 mg/dL.**
4. **After meal = 140 mg/dL.** Two hours after meals.

► Goal values (approximate) <u>**plasma values:**</u>
1. **Fasting =110 ± 20 mg/dL.** Usually first morning. No food or drink for ≥ 8 hours.
2. **Before meals = 110 ± 20 mg/dL.** Essentially the same as fasting.
3. **Bedtime = 130 ± 20 mg/dL.**
4. **After meal = 150 mg/dL.** Two hours after meals.

Monday

Time: _____   Blood Sugar:_____
Time: _____   Blood Sugar:_____
Time: _____   Blood Sugar:_____
Time: _____   Blood Sugar:_____

Tuesday

Time: _____   Blood Sugar:_____
Time: _____   Blood Sugar:_____
Time: _____   Blood Sugar:_____
Time: _____   Blood Sugar:_____

Wednesday, January 1:

Time: _____   Blood Sugar:_____
Time: _____   Blood Sugar:_____
Time: _____   Blood Sugar:_____
Time: _____   Blood Sugar:_____

Thursday, January 2:

Time: _____   Blood Sugar:_____
Time: _____   Blood Sugar:_____
Time: _____   Blood Sugar:_____
Time: _____   Blood Sugar:_____

Friday, January 3:

Time: _____   Blood Sugar:_____
Time: _____   Blood Sugar:_____
Time: _____   Blood Sugar:_____
Time: _____   Blood Sugar:_____

Saturday, January 4:

Time: _____   Blood Sugar:_____
Time: _____   Blood Sugar:_____
Time: _____   Blood Sugar:_____
Time: _____   Blood Sugar:_____

Sunday, January 5:

Time: _____   Blood Sugar:_____
Time: _____   Blood Sugar:_____
Time: _____   Blood Sugar:_____
Time: _____   Blood Sugar:_____

Notes:

Monday, January 6:

Time: _____   Blood Sugar:_____
Time: _____   Blood Sugar:_____
Time: _____   Blood Sugar:_____
Time: _____   Blood Sugar:_____

Tuesday, January 7:

Time: _____   Blood Sugar:_____
Time: _____   Blood Sugar:_____
Time: _____   Blood Sugar:_____
Time: _____   Blood Sugar:_____

Wednesday, January 8:

Time: _____   Blood Sugar:_____
Time: _____   Blood Sugar:_____
Time: _____   Blood Sugar:_____
Time: _____   Blood Sugar:_____

Thursday, January 9:

Time: _____   Blood Sugar:_____
Time: _____   Blood Sugar:_____
Time: _____   Blood Sugar:_____
Time: _____   Blood Sugar:_____

Friday, January 10:

Time: _____   Blood Sugar:_____
Time: _____   Blood Sugar:_____
Time: _____   Blood Sugar:_____
Time: _____   Blood Sugar:_____

Saturday, January 11:

Time: _____   Blood Sugar:_____
Time: _____   Blood Sugar:_____
Time: _____   Blood Sugar:_____
Time: _____   Blood Sugar:_____

Sunday, January 12:

Time: _____   Blood Sugar:_____
Time: _____   Blood Sugar:_____
Time: _____   Blood Sugar:_____
Time: _____   Blood Sugar:_____

Notes:

Monday, January 13:

Time: _____   Blood Sugar:_____
Time: _____   Blood Sugar:_____
Time: _____   Blood Sugar:_____
Time: _____   Blood Sugar:_____

Tuesday, January 14:

Time: _____   Blood Sugar:_____
Time: _____   Blood Sugar:_____
Time: _____   Blood Sugar:_____
Time: _____   Blood Sugar:_____

Wednesday, January 15:

Time: _____   Blood Sugar:_____
Time: _____   Blood Sugar:_____
Time: _____   Blood Sugar:_____
Time: _____   Blood Sugar:_____

Thursday, January 16:

Time: _____   Blood Sugar:_____
Time: _____   Blood Sugar:_____
Time: _____   Blood Sugar:_____
Time: _____   Blood Sugar:_____

Friday, January 17:

Time: _____   Blood Sugar:_____
Time: _____   Blood Sugar:_____
Time: _____   Blood Sugar:_____
Time: _____   Blood Sugar:_____

Saturday, January 18:

Time: _____   Blood Sugar:_____
Time: _____   Blood Sugar:_____
Time: _____   Blood Sugar:_____
Time: _____   Blood Sugar:_____

Sunday, January 19:

Time: _____   Blood Sugar:_____
Time: _____   Blood Sugar:_____
Time: _____   Blood Sugar:_____
Time: _____   Blood Sugar:_____

Notes:

Monday, January 20:

Time: _____ Blood Sugar:_____
Time: _____ Blood Sugar:_____
Time: _____ Blood Sugar:_____
Time: _____ Blood Sugar:_____

Tuesday, January 21:

Time: _____ Blood Sugar:_____
Time: _____ Blood Sugar:_____
Time: _____ Blood Sugar:_____
Time: _____ Blood Sugar:_____

Wednesday, January 22:

Time: _____ Blood Sugar:_____
Time: _____ Blood Sugar:_____
Time: _____ Blood Sugar:_____
Time: _____ Blood Sugar:_____

Thursday, January 23:

Time: _____ Blood Sugar:_____
Time: _____ Blood Sugar:_____
Time: _____ Blood Sugar:_____
Time: _____ Blood Sugar:_____

Friday, January 24:

Time: _____ Blood Sugar:_____
Time: _____ Blood Sugar:_____
Time: _____ Blood Sugar:_____
Time: _____ Blood Sugar:_____

Saturday, January 25:

Time: _____   Blood Sugar:_____
Time: _____   Blood Sugar:_____
Time: _____   Blood Sugar:_____
Time: _____   Blood Sugar:_____

Sunday, January 26:

Time: _____   Blood Sugar:_____
Time: _____   Blood Sugar:_____
Time: _____   Blood Sugar:_____
Time: _____   Blood Sugar:_____

Notes:

Monday, January 27:

Time: _____   Blood Sugar:_____
Time: _____   Blood Sugar:_____
Time: _____   Blood Sugar:_____
Time: _____   Blood Sugar:_____

Tuesday, January 28:

Time: _____   Blood Sugar:_____
Time: _____   Blood Sugar:_____
Time: _____   Blood Sugar:_____
Time: _____   Blood Sugar:_____

Wednesday, January 29:

Time: _____   Blood Sugar:_____
Time: _____   Blood Sugar:_____
Time: _____   Blood Sugar:_____
Time: _____   Blood Sugar:_____

Thursday, January 30:

Time: _____   Blood Sugar:_____
Time: _____   Blood Sugar:_____
Time: _____   Blood Sugar:_____
Time: _____   Blood Sugar:_____

Friday, January 31:

Time: _____   Blood Sugar:_____
Time: _____   Blood Sugar:_____
Time: _____   Blood Sugar:_____
Time: _____   Blood Sugar:_____

Saturday

Time: _____   Blood Sugar:_____
Time: _____   Blood Sugar:_____
Time: _____   Blood Sugar:_____
Time: _____   Blood Sugar:_____

Sunday

Time: _____   Blood Sugar:_____
Time: _____   Blood Sugar:_____
Time: _____   Blood Sugar:_____
Time: _____   Blood Sugar:_____

Notes:

HOME BLOOD SUGAR MONITORING RECORDS

FEBRUARY

▶ Goal values (approximate) <u>**whole blood values:**</u>

1. **Fasting =100 ± 20 mg/dL. Usually first morning.** No food or drink for ≥ 8 hours.

2. **Before meals = 100 ± 20 mg/dL.** Essentially the same as fasting.

3. **Bedtime = 120 ± 20 mg/dL.**

4. **After meal = 140 mg/dL.** Two hours after meals.

▶ Goal values (approximate) <u>**plasma values:**</u>

1. **Fasting =110 ± 20 mg/dL. Usually first morning.** No food or drink for ≥ 8 hours.

2. **Before meals = 110 ± 20 mg/dL.** Essentially the same as fasting.

3. **Bedtime = 130 ± 20 mg/dL.**

4. **After meal = 150 mg/dL.** Two hours after meals.

Monday

Time: _____   Blood Sugar:_____
Time: _____   Blood Sugar:_____
Time: _____   Blood Sugar:_____
Time: _____   Blood Sugar:_____

Tuesday

Time: _____   Blood Sugar:_____
Time: _____   Blood Sugar:_____
Time: _____   Blood Sugar:_____
Time: _____   Blood Sugar:_____

Wednesday

Time: _____   Blood Sugar:_____
Time: _____   Blood Sugar:_____
Time: _____   Blood Sugar:_____
Time: _____   Blood Sugar:_____

Thursday

Time: _____   Blood Sugar:_____
Time: _____   Blood Sugar:_____
Time: _____   Blood Sugar:_____
Time: _____   Blood Sugar:_____

Friday

Time: _____   Blood Sugar:_____
Time: _____   Blood Sugar:_____
Time: _____   Blood Sugar:_____
Time: _____   Blood Sugar:_____

Saturday, February 1:

Time: _____   Blood Sugar:_____
Time: _____   Blood Sugar:_____
Time: _____   Blood Sugar:_____
Time: _____   Blood Sugar:_____

Sunday, February 2:

Time: _____   Blood Sugar:_____
Time: _____   Blood Sugar:_____
Time: _____   Blood Sugar:_____
Time: _____   Blood Sugar:_____

Notes:

Monday, February 3:

Time: _____   Blood Sugar:_____
Time: _____   Blood Sugar:_____
Time: _____   Blood Sugar:_____
Time: _____   Blood Sugar:_____

Tuesday, February 4:

Time: _____   Blood Sugar:_____
Time: _____   Blood Sugar:_____
Time: _____   Blood Sugar:_____
Time: _____   Blood Sugar:_____

Wednesday, February 5:

Time: _____   Blood Sugar:_____
Time: _____   Blood Sugar:_____
Time: _____   Blood Sugar:_____
Time: _____   Blood Sugar:_____

Thursday, February 6:

Time: _____   Blood Sugar:_____
Time: _____   Blood Sugar:_____
Time: _____   Blood Sugar:_____
Time: _____   Blood Sugar:_____

Friday, February 7:

Time: _____   Blood Sugar:_____
Time: _____   Blood Sugar:_____
Time: _____   Blood Sugar:_____
Time: _____   Blood Sugar:_____

Saturday, February 8:

Time: _____   Blood Sugar:_____
Time: _____   Blood Sugar:_____
Time: _____   Blood Sugar:_____
Time: _____   Blood Sugar:_____

Sunday, February 9:

Time: _____   Blood Sugar:_____
Time: _____   Blood Sugar:_____
Time: _____   Blood Sugar:_____
Time: _____   Blood Sugar:_____

Notes:

Monday, February 10:

Time: _____ Blood Sugar:_____
Time: _____ Blood Sugar:_____
Time: _____ Blood Sugar:_____
Time: _____ Blood Sugar:_____

Tuesday, February 11:

Time: _____ Blood Sugar:_____
Time: _____ Blood Sugar:_____
Time: _____ Blood Sugar:_____
Time: _____ Blood Sugar:_____

Wednesday, February 12:

Time: _____ Blood Sugar:_____
Time: _____ Blood Sugar:_____
Time: _____ Blood Sugar:_____
Time: _____ Blood Sugar:_____

Thursday, February 13:

Time: _____ Blood Sugar:_____
Time: _____ Blood Sugar:_____
Time: _____ Blood Sugar:_____
Time: _____ Blood Sugar:_____

Friday, February 14:

Time: _____ Blood Sugar:_____
Time: _____ Blood Sugar:_____
Time: _____ Blood Sugar:_____
Time: _____ Blood Sugar:_____

Saturday, February 15:

Time: _____   Blood Sugar:_____
Time: _____   Blood Sugar:_____
Time: _____   Blood Sugar:_____
Time: _____   Blood Sugar:_____

Sunday, February 16:

Time: _____   Blood Sugar:_____
Time: _____   Blood Sugar:_____
Time: _____   Blood Sugar:_____
Time: _____   Blood Sugar:_____

Notes:

Monday, February 17:

Time: _____ Blood Sugar:_____
Time: _____ Blood Sugar:_____
Time: _____ Blood Sugar:_____
Time: _____ Blood Sugar:_____

Tuesday, February 18:

Time: _____ Blood Sugar:_____
Time: _____ Blood Sugar:_____
Time: _____ Blood Sugar:_____
Time: _____ Blood Sugar:_____

Wednesday, February 19:

Time: _____ Blood Sugar:_____
Time: _____ Blood Sugar:_____
Time: _____ Blood Sugar:_____
Time: _____ Blood Sugar:_____

Thursday, February 20:

Time: _____ Blood Sugar:_____
Time: _____ Blood Sugar:_____
Time: _____ Blood Sugar:_____
Time: _____ Blood Sugar:_____

Friday, February 21:

Time: _____ Blood Sugar:_____
Time: _____ Blood Sugar:_____
Time: _____ Blood Sugar:_____
Time: _____ Blood Sugar:_____

Saturday, February 22:

Time: _____   Blood Sugar:_____
Time: _____   Blood Sugar:_____
Time: _____   Blood Sugar:_____
Time: _____   Blood Sugar:_____

Sunday, February 23:

Time: _____   Blood Sugar:_____
Time: _____   Blood Sugar:_____
Time: _____   Blood Sugar:_____
Time: _____   Blood Sugar:_____

Notes:

Monday, February 24:

Time: _____   Blood Sugar:_____
Time: _____   Blood Sugar:_____
Time: _____   Blood Sugar:_____
Time: _____   Blood Sugar:_____

Tuesday, February 25:

Time: _____   Blood Sugar:_____
Time: _____   Blood Sugar:_____
Time: _____   Blood Sugar:_____
Time: _____   Blood Sugar:_____

Wednesday, February 26:

Time: _____   Blood Sugar:_____
Time: _____   Blood Sugar:_____
Time: _____   Blood Sugar:_____
Time: _____   Blood Sugar:_____

Thursday, February 27:

Time: _____   Blood Sugar:_____
Time: _____   Blood Sugar:_____
Time: _____   Blood Sugar:_____
Time: _____   Blood Sugar:_____

Friday, February 28:

Time: _____   Blood Sugar:_____
Time: _____   Blood Sugar:_____
Time: _____   Blood Sugar:_____
Time: _____   Blood Sugar:_____

Saturday

Time: _____   Blood Sugar:_____
Time: _____   Blood Sugar:_____
Time: _____   Blood Sugar:_____
Time: _____   Blood Sugar:_____

Sunday

Time: _____   Blood Sugar:_____
Time: _____   Blood Sugar:_____
Time: _____   Blood Sugar:_____
Time: _____   Blood Sugar:_____

Notes:

HOME BLOOD SUGAR MONITORING RECORDS

MARCH

▶ Goal values (approximate) <u>**whole blood values:**</u>

1. **Fasting =100 ± 20 mg/dL.** Usually first morning. No food or drink for ≥ 8 hours.

2. **Before meals = 100 ± 20 mg/dL.** Essentially the same as fasting.

3. **Bedtime = 120 ± 20 mg/dL.**

4. **After meal = 140 mg/dL.** Two hours after meals.

▶ Goal values (approximate) <u>**plasma values:**</u>

1. **Fasting =110 ± 20 mg/dL.** Usually first morning. No food or drink for ≥ 8 hours.

2. **Before meals = 110 ± 20 mg/dL.** Essentially the same as fasting.

3. **Bedtime = 130 ± 20 mg/dL.**

4. **After meal = 150 mg/dL.** Two hours after meals.

Monday

Time: _____   Blood Sugar:_____
Time: _____   Blood Sugar:_____
Time: _____   Blood Sugar:_____
Time: _____   Blood Sugar:_____

Tuesday

Time: _____   Blood Sugar:_____
Time: _____   Blood Sugar:_____
Time: _____   Blood Sugar:_____
Time: _____   Blood Sugar:_____

Wednesday

Time: _____   Blood Sugar:_____
Time: _____   Blood Sugar:_____
Time: _____   Blood Sugar:_____
Time: _____   Blood Sugar:_____

Thursday

Time: _____   Blood Sugar:_____
Time: _____   Blood Sugar:_____
Time: _____   Blood Sugar:_____
Time: _____   Blood Sugar:_____

Friday

Time: _____   Blood Sugar:_____
Time: _____   Blood Sugar:_____
Time: _____   Blood Sugar:_____
Time: _____   Blood Sugar:_____

Saturday, March 1:

Time: _____   Blood Sugar:_____
Time: _____   Blood Sugar:_____
Time: _____   Blood Sugar:_____
Time: _____   Blood Sugar:_____

Sunday, March 2:

Time: _____   Blood Sugar:_____
Time: _____   Blood Sugar:_____
Time: _____   Blood Sugar:_____
Time: _____   Blood Sugar:_____

Notes:

Monday, March 3:

Time: _____   Blood Sugar:_____
Time: _____   Blood Sugar:_____
Time: _____   Blood Sugar:_____
Time: _____   Blood Sugar:_____

Tuesday, March 4:

Time: _____   Blood Sugar:_____
Time: _____   Blood Sugar:_____
Time: _____   Blood Sugar:_____
Time: _____   Blood Sugar:_____

Wednesday, March 5:

Time: _____   Blood Sugar:_____
Time: _____   Blood Sugar:_____
Time: _____   Blood Sugar:_____
Time: _____   Blood Sugar:_____

Thursday, March 6:

Time: _____   Blood Sugar:_____
Time: _____   Blood Sugar:_____
Time: _____   Blood Sugar:_____
Time: _____   Blood Sugar:_____

Friday, March 7:

Time: _____   Blood Sugar:_____
Time: _____   Blood Sugar:_____
Time: _____   Blood Sugar:_____
Time: _____   Blood Sugar:_____

Saturday, March 8:

Time: _____   Blood Sugar:_____
Time: _____   Blood Sugar:_____
Time: _____   Blood Sugar:_____
Time: _____   Blood Sugar:_____

Sunday, March 9:

Time: _____   Blood Sugar:_____
Time: _____   Blood Sugar:_____
Time: _____   Blood Sugar:_____
Time: _____   Blood Sugar:_____

Notes:

Monday, March 10:

Time: _____   Blood Sugar:_____
Time: _____   Blood Sugar:_____
Time: _____   Blood Sugar:_____
Time: _____   Blood Sugar:_____

Tuesday, March 11:

Time: _____   Blood Sugar:_____
Time: _____   Blood Sugar:_____
Time: _____   Blood Sugar:_____
Time: _____   Blood Sugar:_____

Wednesday, March 12:

Time: _____   Blood Sugar:_____
Time: _____   Blood Sugar:_____
Time: _____   Blood Sugar:_____
Time: _____   Blood Sugar:_____

Thursday, March 13:

Time: _____   Blood Sugar:_____
Time: _____   Blood Sugar:_____
Time: _____   Blood Sugar:_____
Time: _____   Blood Sugar:_____

Friday, March 14:

Time: _____   Blood Sugar:_____
Time: _____   Blood Sugar:_____
Time: _____   Blood Sugar:_____
Time: _____   Blood Sugar:_____

Saturday, March 15:

Time: _____ Blood Sugar:_____
Time: _____ Blood Sugar:_____
Time: _____ Blood Sugar:_____
Time: _____ Blood Sugar:_____

Sunday, March 16:

Time: _____ Blood Sugar:_____
Time: _____ Blood Sugar:_____
Time: _____ Blood Sugar:_____
Time: _____ Blood Sugar:_____

Notes:

Monday, March 17:

Time: _____ Blood Sugar:_____
Time: _____ Blood Sugar:_____
Time: _____ Blood Sugar:_____
Time: _____ Blood Sugar:_____

Tuesday, March 18:

Time: _____ Blood Sugar:_____
Time: _____ Blood Sugar:_____
Time: _____ Blood Sugar:_____
Time: _____ Blood Sugar:_____

Wednesday, March 19:

Time: _____ Blood Sugar:_____
Time: _____ Blood Sugar:_____
Time: _____ Blood Sugar:_____
Time: _____ Blood Sugar:_____

Thursday, March 20:

Time: _____ Blood Sugar:_____
Time: _____ Blood Sugar:_____
Time: _____ Blood Sugar:_____
Time: _____ Blood Sugar:_____

Friday, March 21:

Time: _____ Blood Sugar:_____
Time: _____ Blood Sugar:_____
Time: _____ Blood Sugar:_____
Time: _____ Blood Sugar:_____

Saturday, March 22:

Time: _____   Blood Sugar:_____
Time: _____   Blood Sugar:_____
Time: _____   Blood Sugar:_____
Time: _____   Blood Sugar:_____

Sunday, March 23:

Time: _____   Blood Sugar:_____
Time: _____   Blood Sugar:_____
Time: _____   Blood Sugar:_____
Time: _____   Blood Sugar:_____

Notes:

Monday, March 24:

Time: _____   Blood Sugar:_____
Time: _____   Blood Sugar:_____
Time: _____   Blood Sugar:_____
Time: _____   Blood Sugar:_____

Tuesday, March 25:

Time: _____   Blood Sugar:_____
Time: _____   Blood Sugar:_____
Time: _____   Blood Sugar:_____
Time: _____   Blood Sugar:_____

Wednesday, March 26:

Time: _____   Blood Sugar:_____
Time: _____   Blood Sugar:_____
Time: _____   Blood Sugar:_____
Time: _____   Blood Sugar:_____

Thursday, March 27:

Time: _____   Blood Sugar:_____
Time: _____   Blood Sugar:_____
Time: _____   Blood Sugar:_____
Time: _____   Blood Sugar:_____

Friday, March 28:

Time: _____   Blood Sugar:_____
Time: _____   Blood Sugar:_____
Time: _____   Blood Sugar:_____
Time: _____   Blood Sugar:_____

Saturday, March 29:

Time: _____   Blood Sugar:_____
Time: _____   Blood Sugar:_____
Time: _____   Blood Sugar:_____
Time: _____   Blood Sugar:_____

Sunday, March 30:

Time: _____   Blood Sugar:_____
Time: _____   Blood Sugar:_____
Time: _____   Blood Sugar:_____
Time: _____   Blood Sugar:_____

Notes:

Monday, March 31:

Time: _____   Blood Sugar:_____
Time: _____   Blood Sugar:_____
Time: _____   Blood Sugar:_____
Time: _____   Blood Sugar:_____

Tuesday

Time: _____   Blood Sugar:_____
Time: _____   Blood Sugar:_____
Time: _____   Blood Sugar:_____
Time: _____   Blood Sugar:_____

Wednesday

Time: _____   Blood Sugar:_____
Time: _____   Blood Sugar:_____
Time: _____   Blood Sugar:_____
Time: _____   Blood Sugar:_____

Thursday

Time: _____   Blood Sugar:_____
Time: _____   Blood Sugar:_____
Time: _____   Blood Sugar:_____
Time: _____   Blood Sugar:_____

Friday

Time: _____   Blood Sugar:_____
Time: _____   Blood Sugar:_____
Time: _____   Blood Sugar:_____
Time: _____   Blood Sugar:_____

Saturday

Time: _____   Blood Sugar:_____
Time: _____   Blood Sugar:_____
Time: _____   Blood Sugar:_____
Time: _____   Blood Sugar:_____

Sunday

Time: _____   Blood Sugar:_____
Time: _____   Blood Sugar:_____
Time: _____   Blood Sugar:_____
Time: _____   Blood Sugar:_____

Notes:

HOME BLOOD SUGAR MONITORING RECORDS

APRIL

▶ Goal values (approximate) <u>**whole blood values:**</u>

1. **Fasting** =100 ± 20 mg/dL. Usually first morning. No food or drink for ≥ 8 hours.

2. **Before meals** = 100 ± 20 mg/dL. Essentially the same as fasting.

3. **Bedtime** = 120 ± 20 mg/dL.

4. **After meal** = 140 mg/dL. Two hours after meals.

▶ Goal values (approximate) <u>**plasma values:**</u>

1. **Fasting** =110 ± 20 mg/dL. Usually first morning. No food or drink for ≥ 8 hours.

2. **Before meals** = 110 ± 20 mg/dL. Essentially the same as fasting.

3. **Bedtime** = 130 ± 20 mg/dL.

4. **After meal** = 150 mg/dL. Two hours after meals.

Monday

Time: _____   Blood Sugar:_____
Time: _____   Blood Sugar:_____
Time: _____   Blood Sugar:_____
Time: _____   Blood Sugar:_____

Tuesday, April 1:

Time: _____   Blood Sugar:_____
Time: _____   Blood Sugar:_____
Time: _____   Blood Sugar:_____
Time: _____   Blood Sugar:_____

Wednesday, April 2:

Time: _____   Blood Sugar:_____
Time: _____   Blood Sugar:_____
Time: _____   Blood Sugar:_____
Time: _____   Blood Sugar:_____

Thursday, April 3:

Time: _____   Blood Sugar:_____
Time: _____   Blood Sugar:_____
Time: _____   Blood Sugar:_____
Time: _____   Blood Sugar:_____

Friday, April 4:

Time: _____   Blood Sugar:_____
Time: _____   Blood Sugar:_____
Time: _____   Blood Sugar:_____
Time: _____   Blood Sugar:_____

Saturday, April 5:

Time: _____   Blood Sugar:_____
Time: _____   Blood Sugar:_____
Time: _____   Blood Sugar:_____
Time: _____   Blood Sugar:_____

Sunday, April 6:

Time: _____   Blood Sugar:_____
Time: _____   Blood Sugar:_____
Time: _____   Blood Sugar:_____
Time: _____   Blood Sugar:_____

Notes:

Monday, April 7:

Time: _____   Blood Sugar:_____
Time: _____   Blood Sugar:_____
Time: _____   Blood Sugar:_____
Time: _____   Blood Sugar:_____

Tuesday, April 8:

Time: _____   Blood Sugar:_____
Time: _____   Blood Sugar:_____
Time: _____   Blood Sugar:_____
Time: _____   Blood Sugar:_____

Wednesday, April 9:

Time: _____   Blood Sugar:_____
Time: _____   Blood Sugar:_____
Time: _____   Blood Sugar:_____
Time: _____   Blood Sugar:_____

Thursday, April 10:

Time: _____   Blood Sugar:_____
Time: _____   Blood Sugar:_____
Time: _____   Blood Sugar:_____
Time: _____   Blood Sugar:_____

Friday, April 11:

Time: _____   Blood Sugar:_____
Time: _____   Blood Sugar:_____
Time: _____   Blood Sugar:_____
Time: _____   Blood Sugar:_____

Saturday, April 12:

Time: _____   Blood Sugar:_____
Time: _____   Blood Sugar:_____
Time: _____   Blood Sugar:_____
Time: _____   Blood Sugar:_____

Sunday, April 13:

Time: _____   Blood Sugar:_____
Time: _____   Blood Sugar:_____
Time: _____   Blood Sugar:_____
Time: _____   Blood Sugar:_____

Notes:

Monday, April 14:

Time: _____   Blood Sugar:_____
Time: _____   Blood Sugar:_____
Time: _____   Blood Sugar:_____
Time: _____   Blood Sugar:_____

Tuesday, April 15:

Time: _____   Blood Sugar:_____
Time: _____   Blood Sugar:_____
Time: _____   Blood Sugar:_____
Time: _____   Blood Sugar:_____

Wednesday, April 16:

Time: _____   Blood Sugar:_____
Time: _____   Blood Sugar:_____
Time: _____   Blood Sugar:_____
Time: _____   Blood Sugar:_____

Thursday, April 17:

Time: _____   Blood Sugar:_____
Time: _____   Blood Sugar:_____
Time: _____   Blood Sugar:_____
Time: _____   Blood Sugar:_____

Friday, April 18:

Time: _____   Blood Sugar:_____
Time: _____   Blood Sugar:_____
Time: _____   Blood Sugar:_____
Time: _____   Blood Sugar:_____

Saturday, April 19:

Time: _____   Blood Sugar:_____
Time: _____   Blood Sugar:_____
Time: _____   Blood Sugar:_____
Time: _____   Blood Sugar:_____

Sunday, April 20:

Time: _____   Blood Sugar:_____
Time: _____   Blood Sugar:_____
Time: _____   Blood Sugar:_____
Time: _____   Blood Sugar:_____

Notes:

Monday, April 21:

Time: _____   Blood Sugar:_____
Time: _____   Blood Sugar:_____
Time: _____   Blood Sugar:_____
Time: _____   Blood Sugar:_____

Tuesday, April 22:

Time: _____   Blood Sugar:_____
Time: _____   Blood Sugar:_____
Time: _____   Blood Sugar:_____
Time: _____   Blood Sugar:_____

Wednesday, April 23:

Time: _____   Blood Sugar:_____
Time: _____   Blood Sugar:_____
Time: _____   Blood Sugar:_____
Time: _____   Blood Sugar:_____

Thursday, April 24:

Time: _____   Blood Sugar:_____
Time: _____   Blood Sugar:_____
Time: _____   Blood Sugar:_____
Time: _____   Blood Sugar:_____

Friday, April 25:

Time: _____   Blood Sugar:_____
Time: _____   Blood Sugar:_____
Time: _____   Blood Sugar:_____
Time: _____   Blood Sugar:_____

Saturday, April 26:

Time: _____ Blood Sugar:_____
Time: _____ Blood Sugar:_____
Time: _____ Blood Sugar:_____
Time: _____ Blood Sugar:_____

Sunday, April 27:

Time: _____ Blood Sugar:_____
Time: _____ Blood Sugar:_____
Time: _____ Blood Sugar:_____
Time: _____ Blood Sugar:_____

Notes:

Monday, April 28:

Time: _____   Blood Sugar:_____
Time: _____   Blood Sugar:_____
Time: _____   Blood Sugar:_____
Time: _____   Blood Sugar:_____

Tuesday, April 29:

Time: _____   Blood Sugar:_____
Time: _____   Blood Sugar:_____
Time: _____   Blood Sugar:_____
Time: _____   Blood Sugar:_____

Wednesday, April 30:

Time: _____   Blood Sugar:_____
Time: _____   Blood Sugar:_____
Time: _____   Blood Sugar:_____
Time: _____   Blood Sugar:_____

Thursday:

Time: _____   Blood Sugar:_____
Time: _____   Blood Sugar:_____
Time: _____   Blood Sugar:_____
Time: _____   Blood Sugar:_____

Friday

Time: _____   Blood Sugar:_____
Time: _____   Blood Sugar:_____
Time: _____   Blood Sugar:_____
Time: _____   Blood Sugar:_____

Saturday

Time: _____   Blood Sugar:_____
Time: _____   Blood Sugar:_____
Time: _____   Blood Sugar:_____
Time: _____   Blood Sugar:_____

Sunday

Time: _____   Blood Sugar:_____
Time: _____   Blood Sugar:_____
Time: _____   Blood Sugar:_____
Time: _____   Blood Sugar:_____

Notes:

HOME BLOOD SUGAR MONITORING RECORDS

MAY

▶ Goal values (approximate) <u>**whole blood values:**</u>

1. **Fasting** =100 ± 20 mg/dL. Usually first morning. No food or drink for ≥ 8 hours.

2. **Before meals** = 100 ± 20 mg/dL. Essentially the same as fasting.

3. **Bedtime** = 120 ± 20 mg/dL.

4. **After meal** = 140 mg/dL. Two hours after meals.

▶ Goal values (approximate) <u>**plasma values:**</u>

1. **Fasting** =110 ± 20 mg/dL. Usually first morning. No food or drink for ≥ 8 hours.

2. **Before meals** = 110 ± 20 mg/dL. Essentially the same as fasting.

3. **Bedtime** = 130 ± 20 mg/dL.

4. **After meal** = 150 mg/dL. Two hours after meals.

Monday

Time: _____   Blood Sugar:_____
Time: _____   Blood Sugar:_____
Time: _____   Blood Sugar:_____
Time: _____   Blood Sugar:_____

Tuesday

Time: _____   Blood Sugar:_____
Time: _____   Blood Sugar:_____
Time: _____   Blood Sugar:_____
Time: _____   Blood Sugar:_____

Wednesday

Time: _____   Blood Sugar:_____
Time: _____   Blood Sugar:_____
Time: _____   Blood Sugar:_____
Time: _____   Blood Sugar:_____

Thursday, May 1:

Time: _____   Blood Sugar:_____
Time: _____   Blood Sugar:_____
Time: _____   Blood Sugar:_____
Time: _____   Blood Sugar:_____

Friday, May 2:

Time: _____   Blood Sugar:_____
Time: _____   Blood Sugar:_____
Time: _____   Blood Sugar:_____
Time: _____   Blood Sugar:_____

Saturday, May 3:

Time: _____   Blood Sugar:_____
Time: _____   Blood Sugar:_____
Time: _____   Blood Sugar:_____
Time: _____   Blood Sugar:_____

Sunday, May 4:

Time: _____   Blood Sugar:_____
Time: _____   Blood Sugar:_____
Time: _____   Blood Sugar:_____
Time: _____   Blood Sugar:_____

Notes:

Monday, May 5:

Time: _____   Blood Sugar:_____
Time: _____   Blood Sugar:_____
Time: _____   Blood Sugar:_____
Time: _____   Blood Sugar:_____

Tuesday, May 6:

Time: _____   Blood Sugar:_____
Time: _____   Blood Sugar:_____
Time: _____   Blood Sugar:_____
Time: _____   Blood Sugar:_____

Wednesday, May 7:

Time: _____   Blood Sugar:_____
Time: _____   Blood Sugar:_____
Time: _____   Blood Sugar:_____
Time: _____   Blood Sugar:_____

Thursday, May 8:

Time: _____   Blood Sugar:_____
Time: _____   Blood Sugar:_____
Time: _____   Blood Sugar:_____
Time: _____   Blood Sugar:_____

Friday, May 9:

Time: _____   Blood Sugar:_____
Time: _____   Blood Sugar:_____
Time: _____   Blood Sugar:_____
Time: _____   Blood Sugar:_____

Saturday, May 10:

Time: _____   Blood Sugar:_____
Time: _____   Blood Sugar:_____
Time: _____   Blood Sugar:_____
Time: _____   Blood Sugar:_____

Sunday, May 11:

Time: _____   Blood Sugar:_____
Time: _____   Blood Sugar:_____
Time: _____   Blood Sugar:_____
Time: _____   Blood Sugar:_____

Notes:

Monday, May 12:

Time: _____　　　　Blood Sugar:_____
Time: _____　　　　Blood Sugar:_____
Time: _____　　　　Blood Sugar:_____
Time: _____　　　　Blood Sugar:_____

Tuesday, May 13:

Time: _____　　　　Blood Sugar:_____
Time: _____　　　　Blood Sugar:_____
Time: _____　　　　Blood Sugar:_____
Time: _____　　　　Blood Sugar:_____

Wednesday, May 14:

Time: _____　　　　Blood Sugar:_____
Time: _____　　　　Blood Sugar:_____
Time: _____　　　　Blood Sugar:_____
Time: _____　　　　Blood Sugar:_____

Thursday, May 15:

Time: _____　　　　Blood Sugar:_____
Time: _____　　　　Blood Sugar:_____
Time: _____　　　　Blood Sugar:_____
Time: _____　　　　Blood Sugar:_____

Friday, May 16:

Time: _____　　　　Blood Sugar:_____
Time: _____　　　　Blood Sugar:_____
Time: _____　　　　Blood Sugar:_____
Time: _____　　　　Blood Sugar:_____

Saturday, May 17:

Time: _____   Blood Sugar:_____
Time: _____   Blood Sugar:_____
Time: _____   Blood Sugar:_____
Time: _____   Blood Sugar:_____

Sunday, May 18:

Time: _____   Blood Sugar:_____
Time: _____   Blood Sugar:_____
Time: _____   Blood Sugar:_____
Time: _____   Blood Sugar:_____

Notes:

Monday, May 19:

Time: _____   Blood Sugar:_____
Time: _____   Blood Sugar:_____
Time: _____   Blood Sugar:_____
Time: _____   Blood Sugar:_____

Tuesday, May 20:

Time: _____   Blood Sugar:_____
Time: _____   Blood Sugar:_____
Time: _____   Blood Sugar:_____
Time: _____   Blood Sugar:_____

Wednesday, May 21:

Time: _____   Blood Sugar:_____
Time: _____   Blood Sugar:_____
Time: _____   Blood Sugar:_____
Time: _____   Blood Sugar:_____

Thursday, May 22:

Time: _____   Blood Sugar:_____
Time: _____   Blood Sugar:_____
Time: _____   Blood Sugar:_____
Time: _____   Blood Sugar:_____

Friday, May 23:

Time: _____   Blood Sugar:_____
Time: _____   Blood Sugar:_____
Time: _____   Blood Sugar:_____
Time: _____   Blood Sugar:_____

Saturday, May 24:

Time: _____ Blood Sugar:_____
Time: _____ Blood Sugar:_____
Time: _____ Blood Sugar:_____
Time: _____ Blood Sugar:_____

Sunday, May 25:

Time: _____ Blood Sugar:_____
Time: _____ Blood Sugar:_____
Time: _____ Blood Sugar:_____
Time: _____ Blood Sugar:_____

Notes:

Monday, May 26:

Time: _____   Blood Sugar:_____
Time: _____   Blood Sugar:_____
Time: _____   Blood Sugar:_____
Time: _____   Blood Sugar:_____

Tuesday, May 27:

Time: _____   Blood Sugar:_____
Time: _____   Blood Sugar:_____
Time: _____   Blood Sugar:_____
Time: _____   Blood Sugar:_____

Wednesday, May 28:

Time: _____   Blood Sugar:_____
Time: _____   Blood Sugar:_____
Time: _____   Blood Sugar:_____
Time: _____   Blood Sugar:_____

Thursday, May 29:

Time: _____   Blood Sugar:_____
Time: _____   Blood Sugar:_____
Time: _____   Blood Sugar:_____
Time: _____   Blood Sugar:_____

Friday, May 30:

Time: _____   Blood Sugar:_____
Time: _____   Blood Sugar:_____
Time: _____   Blood Sugar:_____
Time: _____   Blood Sugar:_____

Saturday, May 31:

Time: _____   Blood Sugar:_____
Time: _____   Blood Sugar:_____
Time: _____   Blood Sugar:_____
Time: _____   Blood Sugar:_____

Sunday

Time: _____   Blood Sugar:_____
Time: _____   Blood Sugar:_____
Time: _____   Blood Sugar:_____
Time: _____   Blood Sugar:_____

Notes:

HOME BLOOD SUGAR MONITORING RECORDS

JUNE

▶ Goal values (approximate) <u>**whole blood values:**</u>

1. **Fasting** =100 ± 20 mg/dL. Usually first morning. No food or drink for ≥ 8 hours.

2. **Before meals** = 100 ± 20 mg/dL. Essentially the same as fasting.

3. **Bedtime** = 120 ± 20 mg/dL.

4. **After meal** = 140 mg/dL. Two hours after meals.

▶ Goal values (approximate) <u>**plasma values:**</u>

1. **Fasting** =110 ± 20 mg/dL. Usually first morning. No food or drink for ≥ 8 hours.

2. **Before meals** = 110 ± 20 mg/dL. Essentially the same as fasting.

3. **Bedtime** = 130 ± 20 mg/dL.

4. **After meal** = 150 mg/dL. Two hours after meals.

Monday

Time: _____   Blood Sugar:_____
Time: _____   Blood Sugar:_____
Time: _____   Blood Sugar:_____
Time: _____   Blood Sugar:_____

Tuesday

Time: _____   Blood Sugar:_____
Time: _____   Blood Sugar:_____
Time: _____   Blood Sugar:_____
Time: _____   Blood Sugar:_____

Wednesday

Time: _____   Blood Sugar:_____
Time: _____   Blood Sugar:_____
Time: _____   Blood Sugar:_____
Time: _____   Blood Sugar:_____

Thursday

Time: _____   Blood Sugar:_____
Time: _____   Blood Sugar:_____
Time: _____   Blood Sugar:_____
Time: _____   Blood Sugar:_____

Friday

Time: _____   Blood Sugar:_____
Time: _____   Blood Sugar:_____
Time: _____   Blood Sugar:_____
Time: _____   Blood Sugar:_____

Saturday

Time: _____   Blood Sugar:_____
Time: _____   Blood Sugar:_____
Time: _____   Blood Sugar:_____
Time: _____   Blood Sugar:_____

Sunday, June 1:

Time: _____   Blood Sugar:_____
Time: _____   Blood Sugar:_____
Time: _____   Blood Sugar:_____
Time: _____   Blood Sugar:_____

Notes:

Monday, June 2:

Time: _____   Blood Sugar:_____
Time: _____   Blood Sugar:_____
Time: _____   Blood Sugar:_____
Time: _____   Blood Sugar:_____

Tuesday, June 3:

Time: _____   Blood Sugar:_____
Time: _____   Blood Sugar:_____
Time: _____   Blood Sugar:_____
Time: _____   Blood Sugar:_____

Wednesday, June 4:

Time: _____   Blood Sugar:_____
Time: _____   Blood Sugar:_____
Time: _____   Blood Sugar:_____
Time: _____   Blood Sugar:_____

Thursday, June 5:

Time: _____   Blood Sugar:_____
Time: _____   Blood Sugar:_____
Time: _____   Blood Sugar:_____
Time: _____   Blood Sugar:_____

Friday, June 6:

Time: _____   Blood Sugar:_____
Time: _____   Blood Sugar:_____
Time: _____   Blood Sugar:_____
Time: _____   Blood Sugar:_____

Saturday, June 7:

Time: _____   Blood Sugar:_____
Time: _____   Blood Sugar:_____
Time: _____   Blood Sugar:_____
Time: _____   Blood Sugar:_____

Sunday, June 8:

Time: _____   Blood Sugar:_____
Time: _____   Blood Sugar:_____
Time: _____   Blood Sugar:_____
Time: _____   Blood Sugar:_____

Notes:

Monday, June 9:

Time: _____   Blood Sugar:_____
Time: _____   Blood Sugar:_____
Time: _____   Blood Sugar:_____
Time: _____   Blood Sugar:_____

Tuesday, June 10:

Time: _____   Blood Sugar:_____
Time: _____   Blood Sugar:_____
Time: _____   Blood Sugar:_____
Time: _____   Blood Sugar:_____

Wednesday, June 11:

Time: _____   Blood Sugar:_____
Time: _____   Blood Sugar:_____
Time: _____   Blood Sugar:_____
Time: _____   Blood Sugar:_____

Thursday, June 12:

Time: _____   Blood Sugar:_____
Time: _____   Blood Sugar:_____
Time: _____   Blood Sugar:_____
Time: _____   Blood Sugar:_____

Friday, June 13:

Time: _____   Blood Sugar:_____
Time: _____   Blood Sugar:_____
Time: _____   Blood Sugar:_____
Time: _____   Blood Sugar:_____

Saturday, June 14:

Time: _____   Blood Sugar:_____
Time: _____   Blood Sugar:_____
Time: _____   Blood Sugar:_____
Time: _____   Blood Sugar:_____

Sunday, June 15:

Time: _____   Blood Sugar:_____
Time: _____   Blood Sugar:_____
Time: _____   Blood Sugar:_____
Time: _____   Blood Sugar:_____

Notes:

Monday, June 16:

Time: _____   Blood Sugar:_____
Time: _____   Blood Sugar:_____
Time: _____   Blood Sugar:_____
Time: _____   Blood Sugar:_____

Tuesday, June 17:

Time: _____   Blood Sugar:_____
Time: _____   Blood Sugar:_____
Time: _____   Blood Sugar:_____
Time: _____   Blood Sugar:_____

Wednesday, June 18:

Time: _____   Blood Sugar:_____
Time: _____   Blood Sugar:_____
Time: _____   Blood Sugar:_____
Time: _____   Blood Sugar:_____

Thursday, June 19:

Time: _____   Blood Sugar:_____
Time: _____   Blood Sugar:_____
Time: _____   Blood Sugar:_____
Time: _____   Blood Sugar:_____

Friday, June 20:

Time: _____   Blood Sugar:_____
Time: _____   Blood Sugar:_____
Time: _____   Blood Sugar:_____
Time: _____   Blood Sugar:_____

Saturday, June 21:

Time: _____   Blood Sugar:_____
Time: _____   Blood Sugar:_____
Time: _____   Blood Sugar:_____
Time: _____   Blood Sugar:_____

Sunday, June 22:

Time: _____   Blood Sugar:_____
Time: _____   Blood Sugar:_____
Time: _____   Blood Sugar:_____
Time: _____   Blood Sugar:_____

Notes:

Monday, June 23:

Time: _____ Blood Sugar:_____
Time: _____ Blood Sugar:_____
Time: _____ Blood Sugar:_____
Time: _____ Blood Sugar:_____

Tuesday, June 24:

Time: _____ Blood Sugar:_____
Time: _____ Blood Sugar:_____
Time: _____ Blood Sugar:_____
Time: _____ Blood Sugar:_____

Wednesday, June 25:

Time: _____ Blood Sugar:_____
Time: _____ Blood Sugar:_____
Time: _____ Blood Sugar:_____
Time: _____ Blood Sugar:_____

Thursday, June 26:

Time: _____ Blood Sugar:_____
Time: _____ Blood Sugar:_____
Time: _____ Blood Sugar:_____
Time: _____ Blood Sugar:_____

Friday, June 27:

Time: _____ Blood Sugar:_____
Time: _____ Blood Sugar:_____
Time: _____ Blood Sugar:_____
Time: _____ Blood Sugar:_____

Saturday, June 28:

Time: _____   Blood Sugar:_____
Time: _____   Blood Sugar:_____
Time: _____   Blood Sugar:_____
Time: _____   Blood Sugar:_____

Sunday, June 29:

Time: _____   Blood Sugar:_____
Time: _____   Blood Sugar:_____
Time: _____   Blood Sugar:_____
Time: _____   Blood Sugar:_____

Notes:

Monday, June 30:

Time: _____   Blood Sugar:_____
Time: _____   Blood Sugar:_____
Time: _____   Blood Sugar:_____
Time: _____   Blood Sugar:_____

Tuesday

Time: _____   Blood Sugar:_____
Time: _____   Blood Sugar:_____
Time: _____   Blood Sugar:_____
Time: _____   Blood Sugar:_____

Wednesday

Time: _____   Blood Sugar:_____
Time: _____   Blood Sugar:_____
Time: _____   Blood Sugar:_____
Time: _____   Blood Sugar:_____

Thursday

Time: _____   Blood Sugar:_____
Time: _____   Blood Sugar:_____
Time: _____   Blood Sugar:_____
Time: _____   Blood Sugar:_____

Friday

Time: _____   Blood Sugar:_____
Time: _____   Blood Sugar:_____
Time: _____   Blood Sugar:_____
Time: _____   Blood Sugar:_____

Saturday

Time: _____   Blood Sugar:_____
Time: _____   Blood Sugar:_____
Time: _____   Blood Sugar:_____
Time: _____   Blood Sugar:_____

Sunday

Time: _____   Blood Sugar:_____
Time: _____   Blood Sugar:_____
Time: _____   Blood Sugar:_____
Time: _____   Blood Sugar:_____

Notes:

HOME BLOOD SUGAR MONITORING RECORDS

JULY

▶ Goal values (approximate) <u>**whole blood values:**</u>

1. **Fasting** =**100 ± 20 mg/dL.** Usually first morning. No food or drink for ≥ 8 hours.

2. **Before meals = 100 ± 20 mg/dL.** Essentially the same as fasting.

3. **Bedtime = 120 ± 20 mg/dL.**

4. **After meal = 140 mg/dL.** Two hours after meals.

▶ Goal values (approximate) <u>**plasma values:**</u>

1. **Fasting** =**110 ± 20 mg/dL.** Usually first morning. No food or drink for ≥ 8 hours.

2. **Before meals = 110 ± 20 mg/dL.** Essentially the same as fasting.

3. **Bedtime = 130 ± 20 mg/dL.**

4. **After meal = 150 mg/dL.** Two hours after meals.

Monday

Time: _____   Blood Sugar:_____
Time: _____   Blood Sugar:_____
Time: _____   Blood Sugar:_____
Time: _____   Blood Sugar:_____

Tuesday, July 1:

Time: _____   Blood Sugar:_____
Time: _____   Blood Sugar:_____
Time: _____   Blood Sugar:_____
Time: _____   Blood Sugar:_____

Wednesday, July 2:

Time: _____   Blood Sugar:_____
Time: _____   Blood Sugar:_____
Time: _____   Blood Sugar:_____
Time: _____   Blood Sugar:_____

Thursday, July 3:

Time: _____   Blood Sugar:_____
Time: _____   Blood Sugar:_____
Time: _____   Blood Sugar:_____
Time: _____   Blood Sugar:_____

Friday, July 4:

Time: _____   Blood Sugar:_____
Time: _____   Blood Sugar:_____
Time: _____   Blood Sugar:_____
Time: _____   Blood Sugar:_____

Saturday, July 5:

Time: _____   Blood Sugar:_____
Time: _____   Blood Sugar:_____
Time: _____   Blood Sugar:_____
Time: _____   Blood Sugar:_____

Sunday, July 6:

Time: _____   Blood Sugar:_____
Time: _____   Blood Sugar:_____
Time: _____   Blood Sugar:_____
Time: _____   Blood Sugar:_____

Notes:

Monday, July 7:

Time: _____   Blood Sugar:_____
Time: _____   Blood Sugar:_____
Time: _____   Blood Sugar:_____
Time: _____   Blood Sugar:_____

Tuesday, July 8:

Time: _____   Blood Sugar:_____
Time: _____   Blood Sugar:_____
Time: _____   Blood Sugar:_____
Time: _____   Blood Sugar:_____

Wednesday, July 9:

Time: _____   Blood Sugar:_____
Time: _____   Blood Sugar:_____
Time: _____   Blood Sugar:_____
Time: _____   Blood Sugar:_____

Thursday, July 10:

Time: _____   Blood Sugar:_____
Time: _____   Blood Sugar:_____
Time: _____   Blood Sugar:_____
Time: _____   Blood Sugar:_____

Friday, July 11:

Time: _____   Blood Sugar:_____
Time: _____   Blood Sugar:_____
Time: _____   Blood Sugar:_____
Time: _____   Blood Sugar:_____

Saturday, July 12:

Time: _____   Blood Sugar:_____
Time: _____   Blood Sugar:_____
Time: _____   Blood Sugar:_____
Time: _____   Blood Sugar:_____

Sunday, July 13:

Time: _____   Blood Sugar:_____
Time: _____   Blood Sugar:_____
Time: _____   Blood Sugar:_____
Time: _____   Blood Sugar:_____

Notes:

Monday, July 14:

Time: _____   Blood Sugar:_____
Time: _____   Blood Sugar:_____
Time: _____   Blood Sugar:_____
Time: _____   Blood Sugar:_____

Tuesday, July 15:

Time: _____   Blood Sugar:_____
Time: _____   Blood Sugar:_____
Time: _____   Blood Sugar:_____
Time: _____   Blood Sugar:_____

Wednesday, July 16:

Time: _____   Blood Sugar:_____
Time: _____   Blood Sugar:_____
Time: _____   Blood Sugar:_____
Time: _____   Blood Sugar:_____

Thursday, July 17:

Time: _____   Blood Sugar:_____
Time: _____   Blood Sugar:_____
Time: _____   Blood Sugar:_____
Time: _____   Blood Sugar:_____

Friday, July 18:

Time: _____   Blood Sugar:_____
Time: _____   Blood Sugar:_____
Time: _____   Blood Sugar:_____
Time: _____   Blood Sugar:_____

Saturday, July 19:

Time: _____   Blood Sugar:_____
Time: _____   Blood Sugar:_____
Time: _____   Blood Sugar:_____
Time: _____   Blood Sugar:_____

Sunday, July 20:

Time: _____   Blood Sugar:_____
Time: _____   Blood Sugar:_____
Time: _____   Blood Sugar:_____
Time: _____   Blood Sugar:_____

Notes:

Monday, July 21:

Time: _____   Blood Sugar:_____

Time: _____   Blood Sugar:_____

Time: _____   Blood Sugar:_____

Time: _____   Blood Sugar:_____

Tuesday, July 22:

Time: _____   Blood Sugar:_____

Time: _____   Blood Sugar:_____

Time: _____   Blood Sugar:_____

Time: _____   Blood Sugar:_____

Wednesday, July 23:

Time: _____   Blood Sugar:_____

Time: _____   Blood Sugar:_____

Time: _____   Blood Sugar:_____

Time: _____   Blood Sugar:_____

Thursday, July 24:

Time: _____   Blood Sugar:_____

Time: _____   Blood Sugar:_____

Time: _____   Blood Sugar:_____

Time: _____   Blood Sugar:_____

Friday, July 25:

Time: _____   Blood Sugar:_____

Time: _____   Blood Sugar:_____

Time: _____   Blood Sugar:_____

Time: _____   Blood Sugar:_____

Saturday, July 26:

Time: _____   Blood Sugar:_____
Time: _____   Blood Sugar:_____
Time: _____   Blood Sugar:_____
Time: _____   Blood Sugar:_____

Sunday, July 27:

Time: _____   Blood Sugar:_____
Time: _____   Blood Sugar:_____
Time: _____   Blood Sugar:_____
Time: _____   Blood Sugar:_____

Notes:

Monday, July 28:

Time: _____   Blood Sugar:_____
Time: _____   Blood Sugar:_____
Time: _____   Blood Sugar:_____
Time: _____   Blood Sugar:_____

Tuesday, July 29:

Time: _____   Blood Sugar:_____
Time: _____   Blood Sugar:_____
Time: _____   Blood Sugar:_____
Time: _____   Blood Sugar:_____

Wednesday, July 30:

Time: _____   Blood Sugar:_____
Time: _____   Blood Sugar:_____
Time: _____   Blood Sugar:_____
Time: _____   Blood Sugar:_____

Thursday, July 31:

Time: _____   Blood Sugar:_____
Time: _____   Blood Sugar:_____
Time: _____   Blood Sugar:_____
Time: _____   Blood Sugar:_____

Friday

Time: _____   Blood Sugar:_____
Time: _____   Blood Sugar:_____
Time: _____   Blood Sugar:_____
Time: _____   Blood Sugar:_____

Saturday

Time: _____   Blood Sugar:_____
Time: _____   Blood Sugar:_____
Time: _____   Blood Sugar:_____
Time: _____   Blood Sugar:_____

Sunday

Time: _____   Blood Sugar:_____
Time: _____   Blood Sugar:_____
Time: _____   Blood Sugar:_____
Time: _____   Blood Sugar:_____

Notes:

HOME BLOOD SUGAR MONITORING RECORDS

AUGUST

▶ Goal values (approximate) **whole blood values:**

1. **Fasting =100 ± 20 mg/dL.** Usually first morning. No food or drink for ≥ 8 hours.

2. **Before meals = 100 ± 20 mg/dL.** Essentially the same as fasting.

3. **Bedtime = 120 ± 20 mg/dL.**

4. **After meal = 140 mg/dL.** Two hours after meals.

▶ Goal values (approximate) **plasma values:**

1. **Fasting =110 ± 20 mg/dL.** Usually first morning. No food or drink for ≥ 8 hours.

2. **Before meals = 110 ± 20 mg/dL.** Essentially the same as fasting.

3. **Bedtime = 130 ± 20 mg/dL.**

4. **After meal = 150 mg/dL.** Two hours after meals.

Monday

Time: _____　　Blood Sugar:_____
Time: _____　　Blood Sugar:_____
Time: _____　　Blood Sugar:_____
Time: _____　　Blood Sugar:_____

Tuesday

Time: _____　　Blood Sugar:_____
Time: _____　　Blood Sugar:_____
Time: _____　　Blood Sugar:_____
Time: _____　　Blood Sugar:_____

Wednesday

Time: _____　　Blood Sugar:_____
Time: _____　　Blood Sugar:_____
Time: _____　　Blood Sugar:_____
Time: _____　　Blood Sugar:_____

Thursday

Time: _____　　Blood Sugar:_____
Time: _____　　Blood Sugar:_____
Time: _____　　Blood Sugar:_____
Time: _____　　Blood Sugar:_____

Friday, August 1:

Time: _____　　Blood Sugar:_____
Time: _____　　Blood Sugar:_____
Time: _____　　Blood Sugar:_____
Time: _____　　Blood Sugar:_____

Saturday, August 2:

Time: _____ Blood Sugar:_____
Time: _____ Blood Sugar:_____
Time: _____ Blood Sugar:_____
Time: _____ Blood Sugar:_____

Sunday, August 3:

Time: _____ Blood Sugar:_____
Time: _____ Blood Sugar:_____
Time: _____ Blood Sugar:_____
Time: _____ Blood Sugar:_____

Notes:

Monday, August 4:

Time: _____   Blood Sugar:_____
Time: _____   Blood Sugar:_____
Time: _____   Blood Sugar:_____
Time: _____   Blood Sugar:_____

Tuesday, August 5:

Time: _____   Blood Sugar:_____
Time: _____   Blood Sugar:_____
Time: _____   Blood Sugar:_____
Time: _____   Blood Sugar:_____

Wednesday, August 6:

Time: _____   Blood Sugar:_____
Time: _____   Blood Sugar:_____
Time: _____   Blood Sugar:_____
Time: _____   Blood Sugar:_____

Thursday, August 7:

Time: _____   Blood Sugar:_____
Time: _____   Blood Sugar:_____
Time: _____   Blood Sugar:_____
Time: _____   Blood Sugar:_____

Friday, August 8:

Time: _____   Blood Sugar:_____
Time: _____   Blood Sugar:_____
Time: _____   Blood Sugar:_____
Time: _____   Blood Sugar:_____

Saturday, August 9:

Time: _____   Blood Sugar:_____

Time: _____   Blood Sugar:_____

Time: _____   Blood Sugar:_____

Time: _____   Blood Sugar:_____

Sunday, August 10:

Time: _____   Blood Sugar:_____

Time: _____   Blood Sugar:_____

Time: _____   Blood Sugar:_____

Time: _____   Blood Sugar:_____

Notes:

Monday, August 11:

Time: _____   Blood Sugar:_____
Time: _____   Blood Sugar:_____
Time: _____   Blood Sugar:_____
Time: _____   Blood Sugar:_____

Tuesday, August 12:

Time: _____   Blood Sugar:_____
Time: _____   Blood Sugar:_____
Time: _____   Blood Sugar:_____
Time: _____   Blood Sugar:_____

Wednesday, August 13:

Time: _____   Blood Sugar:_____
Time: _____   Blood Sugar:_____
Time: _____   Blood Sugar:_____
Time: _____   Blood Sugar:_____

Thursday, August 14:

Time: _____   Blood Sugar:_____
Time: _____   Blood Sugar:_____
Time: _____   Blood Sugar:_____
Time: _____   Blood Sugar:_____

Friday, August 15:

Time: _____   Blood Sugar:_____
Time: _____   Blood Sugar:_____
Time: _____   Blood Sugar:_____
Time: _____   Blood Sugar:_____

Saturday, August 16:

Time: _____ Blood Sugar:_____
Time: _____ Blood Sugar:_____
Time: _____ Blood Sugar:_____
Time: _____ Blood Sugar:_____

Sunday, August 17:

Time: _____ Blood Sugar:_____
Time: _____ Blood Sugar:_____
Time: _____ Blood Sugar:_____
Time: _____ Blood Sugar:_____

Notes:

Monday, August 18:

Time: _____   Blood Sugar:_____
Time: _____   Blood Sugar:_____
Time: _____   Blood Sugar:_____
Time: _____   Blood Sugar:_____

Tuesday, August 19:

Time: _____   Blood Sugar:_____
Time: _____   Blood Sugar:_____
Time: _____   Blood Sugar:_____
Time: _____   Blood Sugar:_____

Wednesday, August 20:

Time: _____   Blood Sugar:_____
Time: _____   Blood Sugar:_____
Time: _____   Blood Sugar:_____
Time: _____   Blood Sugar:_____

Thursday, August 21:

Time: _____   Blood Sugar:_____
Time: _____   Blood Sugar:_____
Time: _____   Blood Sugar:_____
Time: _____   Blood Sugar:_____

Friday, August 22:

Time: _____   Blood Sugar:_____
Time: _____   Blood Sugar:_____
Time: _____   Blood Sugar:_____
Time: _____   Blood Sugar:_____

Saturday, August 23:

Time: _____   Blood Sugar:_____
Time: _____   Blood Sugar:_____
Time: _____   Blood Sugar:_____
Time: _____   Blood Sugar:_____

Sunday, August 24:

Time: _____   Blood Sugar:_____
Time: _____   Blood Sugar:_____
Time: _____   Blood Sugar:_____
Time: _____   Blood Sugar:_____

Notes:

Monday, August 25:

Time: _____   Blood Sugar:_____
Time: _____   Blood Sugar:_____
Time: _____   Blood Sugar:_____
Time: _____   Blood Sugar:_____

Tuesday, August 26:

Time: _____   Blood Sugar:_____
Time: _____   Blood Sugar:_____
Time: _____   Blood Sugar:_____
Time: _____   Blood Sugar:_____

Wednesday, August 27:

Time: _____   Blood Sugar:_____
Time: _____   Blood Sugar:_____
Time: _____   Blood Sugar:_____
Time: _____   Blood Sugar:_____

Thursday, August 28:

Time: _____   Blood Sugar:_____
Time: _____   Blood Sugar:_____
Time: _____   Blood Sugar:_____
Time: _____   Blood Sugar:_____

Friday, August 29:

Time: _____   Blood Sugar:_____
Time: _____   Blood Sugar:_____
Time: _____   Blood Sugar:_____
Time: _____   Blood Sugar:_____

Saturday, August 30:

Time: _____   Blood Sugar:_____
Time: _____   Blood Sugar:_____
Time: _____   Blood Sugar:_____
Time: _____   Blood Sugar:_____

Sunday, August 31:

Time: _____   Blood Sugar:_____
Time: _____   Blood Sugar:_____
Time: _____   Blood Sugar:_____
Time: _____   Blood Sugar:_____

Notes:

HOME BLOOD SUGAR MONITORING RECORDS

SEPTEMBER

▶ Goal values (approximate) <u>**whole blood values:**</u>

1. **Fasting** =100 ± 20 mg/dL. Usually first morning. No food or drink for ≥ 8 hours.
2. **Before meals** = 100 ± 20 mg/dL. Essentially the same as fasting.
3. **Bedtime** = 120 ± 20 mg/dL.
4. **After meal** = 140 mg/dL. Two hours after meals.

▶ Goal values (approximate) <u>**plasma values:**</u>

1. **Fasting** =110 ± 20 mg/dL. Usually first morning. No food or drink for ≥ 8 hours.
2. **Before meals** = 110 ± 20 mg/dL. Essentially the same as fasting.
3. **Bedtime** = 130 ± 20 mg/dL.
4. **After meal** = 150 mg/dL. Two hours after meals.

Monday, September 1:

Time: _____   Blood Sugar:_____
Time: _____   Blood Sugar:_____
Time: _____   Blood Sugar:_____
Time: _____   Blood Sugar:_____

Tuesday, September 2:

Time: _____   Blood Sugar:_____
Time: _____   Blood Sugar:_____
Time: _____   Blood Sugar:_____
Time: _____   Blood Sugar:_____

Wednesday, September 3:

Time: _____   Blood Sugar:_____
Time: _____   Blood Sugar:_____
Time: _____   Blood Sugar:_____
Time: _____   Blood Sugar:_____

Thursday, September 4:

Time: _____   Blood Sugar:_____
Time: _____   Blood Sugar:_____
Time: _____   Blood Sugar:_____
Time: _____   Blood Sugar:_____

Friday, September 5:

Time: _____   Blood Sugar:_____
Time: _____   Blood Sugar:_____
Time: _____   Blood Sugar:_____
Time: _____   Blood Sugar:_____

Saturday, September 6:

Time: _____   Blood Sugar:_____
Time: _____   Blood Sugar:_____
Time: _____   Blood Sugar:_____
Time: _____   Blood Sugar:_____

Sunday, September 7:

Time: _____   Blood Sugar:_____
Time: _____   Blood Sugar:_____
Time: _____   Blood Sugar:_____
Time: _____   Blood Sugar:_____

Notes:

Monday, September 8:

Time: _____   Blood Sugar:_____
Time: _____   Blood Sugar:_____
Time: _____   Blood Sugar:_____
Time: _____   Blood Sugar:_____

Tuesday, September 9:

Time: _____   Blood Sugar:_____
Time: _____   Blood Sugar:_____
Time: _____   Blood Sugar:_____
Time: _____   Blood Sugar:_____

Wednesday, September 10:

Time: _____   Blood Sugar:_____
Time: _____   Blood Sugar:_____
Time: _____   Blood Sugar:_____
Time: _____   Blood Sugar:_____

Thursday, September 11:

Time: _____   Blood Sugar:_____
Time: _____   Blood Sugar:_____
Time: _____   Blood Sugar:_____
Time: _____   Blood Sugar:_____

Friday, September 12:

Time: _____   Blood Sugar:_____
Time: _____   Blood Sugar:_____
Time: _____   Blood Sugar:_____
Time: _____   Blood Sugar:_____

Saturday, September 13:

Time: _____ Blood Sugar:_____
Time: _____ Blood Sugar:_____
Time: _____ Blood Sugar:_____
Time: _____ Blood Sugar:_____

Sunday, September 14:

Time: _____ Blood Sugar:_____
Time: _____ Blood Sugar:_____
Time: _____ Blood Sugar:_____
Time: _____ Blood Sugar:_____

Notes:

Monday, September 15:

Time: _____   Blood Sugar:_____
Time: _____   Blood Sugar:_____
Time: _____   Blood Sugar:_____
Time: _____   Blood Sugar:_____

Tuesday, September 16:

Time: _____   Blood Sugar:_____
Time: _____   Blood Sugar:_____
Time: _____   Blood Sugar:_____
Time: _____   Blood Sugar:_____

Wednesday, September 17:

Time: _____   Blood Sugar:_____
Time: _____   Blood Sugar:_____
Time: _____   Blood Sugar:_____
Time: _____   Blood Sugar:_____

Thursday, September 18:

Time: _____   Blood Sugar:_____
Time: _____   Blood Sugar:_____
Time: _____   Blood Sugar:_____
Time: _____   Blood Sugar:_____

Friday, September 19:

Time: _____   Blood Sugar:_____
Time: _____   Blood Sugar:_____
Time: _____   Blood Sugar:_____
Time: _____   Blood Sugar:_____

Saturday, September 20:

Time: _____ Blood Sugar:_____
Time: _____ Blood Sugar:_____
Time: _____ Blood Sugar:_____
Time: _____ Blood Sugar:_____

Sunday, September 21:

Time: _____ Blood Sugar:_____
Time: _____ Blood Sugar:_____
Time: _____ Blood Sugar:_____
Time: _____ Blood Sugar:_____

Notes:

Monday, September 22:

Time: _____   Blood Sugar:_____
Time: _____   Blood Sugar:_____
Time: _____   Blood Sugar:_____
Time: _____   Blood Sugar:_____

Tuesday, September 23:

Time: _____   Blood Sugar:_____
Time: _____   Blood Sugar:_____
Time: _____   Blood Sugar:_____
Time: _____   Blood Sugar:_____

Wednesday, September 24:

Time: _____   Blood Sugar:_____
Time: _____   Blood Sugar:_____
Time: _____   Blood Sugar:_____
Time: _____   Blood Sugar:_____

Thursday, September 25:

Time: _____   Blood Sugar:_____
Time: _____   Blood Sugar:_____
Time: _____   Blood Sugar:_____
Time: _____   Blood Sugar:_____

Friday, September 26:

Time: _____   Blood Sugar:_____
Time: _____   Blood Sugar:_____
Time: _____   Blood Sugar:_____
Time: _____   Blood Sugar:_____

Saturday, September 27:

Time: _____   Blood Sugar:_____
Time: _____   Blood Sugar:_____
Time: _____   Blood Sugar:_____
Time: _____   Blood Sugar:_____

Sunday, September 28:

Time: _____   Blood Sugar:_____
Time: _____   Blood Sugar:_____
Time: _____   Blood Sugar:_____
Time: _____   Blood Sugar:_____

Notes:

Monday, September 29:

Time: _____   Blood Sugar:_____
Time: _____   Blood Sugar:_____
Time: _____   Blood Sugar:_____
Time: _____   Blood Sugar:_____

Tuesday, September 30:

Time: _____   Blood Sugar:_____
Time: _____   Blood Sugar:_____
Time: _____   Blood Sugar:_____
Time: _____   Blood Sugar:_____

Wednesday

Time: _____   Blood Sugar:_____
Time: _____   Blood Sugar:_____
Time: _____   Blood Sugar:_____
Time: _____   Blood Sugar:_____

Thursday

Time: _____   Blood Sugar:_____
Time: _____   Blood Sugar:_____
Time: _____   Blood Sugar:_____
Time: _____   Blood Sugar:_____

Friday

Time: _____   Blood Sugar:_____
Time: _____   Blood Sugar:_____
Time: _____   Blood Sugar:_____
Time: _____   Blood Sugar:_____

Saturday

Time: _____   Blood Sugar:_____
Time: _____   Blood Sugar:_____
Time: _____   Blood Sugar:_____
Time: _____   Blood Sugar:_____

Sunday

Time: _____   Blood Sugar:_____
Time: _____   Blood Sugar:_____
Time: _____   Blood Sugar:_____
Time: _____   Blood Sugar:_____

Notes:

HOME BLOOD SUGAR MONITORING RECORDS

OCTOBER

▶ Goal values (approximate) <u>**whole blood values:**</u>

1. **Fasting =100 ± 20 mg/dL.** Usually first morning. No food or drink for ≥ 8 hours.

2. **Before meals = 100 ± 20 mg/dL.** Essentially the same as fasting.

3. **Bedtime = 120 ± 20 mg/dL.**

4. **After meal = 140 mg/dL.** Two hours after meals.

▶ Goal values (approximate) <u>**plasma values:**</u>

1. **Fasting =110 ± 20 mg/dL.** Usually first morning. No food or drink for ≥ 8 hours.

2. **Before meals = 110 ± 20 mg/dL.** Essentially the same as fasting.

3. **Bedtime = 130 ± 20 mg/dL.**

4. **After meal = 150 mg/dL.** Two hours after meals.

Monday

Time: _____   Blood Sugar:_____
Time: _____   Blood Sugar:_____
Time: _____   Blood Sugar:_____
Time: _____   Blood Sugar:_____

Tuesday

Time: _____   Blood Sugar:_____
Time: _____   Blood Sugar:_____
Time: _____   Blood Sugar:_____
Time: _____   Blood Sugar:_____

Wednesday, October 1:

Time: _____   Blood Sugar:_____
Time: _____   Blood Sugar:_____
Time: _____   Blood Sugar:_____
Time: _____   Blood Sugar:_____

Thursday, October 2:

Time: _____   Blood Sugar:_____
Time: _____   Blood Sugar:_____
Time: _____   Blood Sugar:_____
Time: _____   Blood Sugar:_____

Friday, October 3:

Time: _____   Blood Sugar:_____
Time: _____   Blood Sugar:_____
Time: _____   Blood Sugar:_____
Time: _____   Blood Sugar:_____

Saturday, October 4:

Time: _____   Blood Sugar:_____
Time: _____   Blood Sugar:_____
Time: _____   Blood Sugar:_____
Time: _____   Blood Sugar:_____

Sunday, October 5:

Time: _____   Blood Sugar:_____
Time: _____   Blood Sugar:_____
Time: _____   Blood Sugar:_____
Time: _____   Blood Sugar:_____

Notes:

Monday, October 6:

Time: _____   Blood Sugar:_____
Time: _____   Blood Sugar:_____
Time: _____   Blood Sugar:_____
Time: _____   Blood Sugar:_____

Tuesday, October 7:

Time: _____   Blood Sugar:_____
Time: _____   Blood Sugar:_____
Time: _____   Blood Sugar:_____
Time: _____   Blood Sugar:_____

Wednesday, October 8:

Time: _____   Blood Sugar:_____
Time: _____   Blood Sugar:_____
Time: _____   Blood Sugar:_____
Time: _____   Blood Sugar:_____

Thursday, October 9:

Time: _____   Blood Sugar:_____
Time: _____   Blood Sugar:_____
Time: _____   Blood Sugar:_____
Time: _____   Blood Sugar:_____

Friday, October 10:

Time: _____   Blood Sugar:_____
Time: _____   Blood Sugar:_____
Time: _____   Blood Sugar:_____
Time: _____   Blood Sugar:_____

Saturday, October 11:

Time: _____   Blood Sugar:_____
Time: _____   Blood Sugar:_____
Time: _____   Blood Sugar:_____
Time: _____   Blood Sugar:_____

Sunday, October 12:

Time: _____   Blood Sugar:_____
Time: _____   Blood Sugar:_____
Time: _____   Blood Sugar:_____
Time: _____   Blood Sugar:_____

Notes:

Monday, October 13:

Time: _____   Blood Sugar:_____
Time: _____   Blood Sugar:_____
Time: _____   Blood Sugar:_____
Time: _____   Blood Sugar:_____

Tuesday, October 14:

Time: _____   Blood Sugar:_____
Time: _____   Blood Sugar:_____
Time: _____   Blood Sugar:_____
Time: _____   Blood Sugar:_____

Wednesday, October 15:

Time: _____   Blood Sugar:_____
Time: _____   Blood Sugar:_____
Time: _____   Blood Sugar:_____
Time: _____   Blood Sugar:_____

Thursday, October 16:

Time: _____   Blood Sugar:_____
Time: _____   Blood Sugar:_____
Time: _____   Blood Sugar:_____
Time: _____   Blood Sugar:_____

Friday, October 17:

Time: _____   Blood Sugar:_____
Time: _____   Blood Sugar:_____
Time: _____   Blood Sugar:_____
Time: _____   Blood Sugar:_____

Saturday, October 18:

Time: _____   Blood Sugar:_____
Time: _____   Blood Sugar:_____
Time: _____   Blood Sugar:_____
Time: _____   Blood Sugar:_____

Sunday, October 19:

Time: _____   Blood Sugar:_____
Time: _____   Blood Sugar:_____
Time: _____   Blood Sugar:_____
Time: _____   Blood Sugar:_____

Notes:

Monday, October 20:

Time: _____   Blood Sugar:_____
Time: _____   Blood Sugar:_____
Time: _____   Blood Sugar:_____
Time: _____   Blood Sugar:_____

Tuesday, October 21:

Time: _____   Blood Sugar:_____
Time: _____   Blood Sugar:_____
Time: _____   Blood Sugar:_____
Time: _____   Blood Sugar:_____

Wednesday, October 22:

Time: _____   Blood Sugar:_____
Time: _____   Blood Sugar:_____
Time: _____   Blood Sugar:_____
Time: _____   Blood Sugar:_____

Thursday, October 23:

Time: _____   Blood Sugar:_____
Time: _____   Blood Sugar:_____
Time: _____   Blood Sugar:_____
Time: _____   Blood Sugar:_____

Friday, October 24:

Time: _____   Blood Sugar:_____
Time: _____   Blood Sugar:_____
Time: _____   Blood Sugar:_____
Time: _____   Blood Sugar:_____

Saturday, October 25:

Time: _____   Blood Sugar:_____
Time: _____   Blood Sugar:_____
Time: _____   Blood Sugar:_____
Time: _____   Blood Sugar:_____

Sunday, October 26:

Time: _____   Blood Sugar:_____
Time: _____   Blood Sugar:_____
Time: _____   Blood Sugar:_____
Time: _____   Blood Sugar:_____

Notes:

Monday, October 27:

Time: _____   Blood Sugar:_____
Time: _____   Blood Sugar:_____
Time: _____   Blood Sugar:_____
Time: _____   Blood Sugar:_____

Tuesday, October 28:

Time: _____   Blood Sugar:_____
Time: _____   Blood Sugar:_____
Time: _____   Blood Sugar:_____
Time: _____   Blood Sugar:_____

Wednesday, October 29:

Time: _____   Blood Sugar:_____
Time: _____   Blood Sugar:_____
Time: _____   Blood Sugar:_____
Time: _____   Blood Sugar:_____

Thursday, October 30:

Time: _____   Blood Sugar:_____
Time: _____   Blood Sugar:_____
Time: _____   Blood Sugar:_____
Time: _____   Blood Sugar:_____

Friday, October 31:

Time: _____   Blood Sugar:_____
Time: _____   Blood Sugar:_____
Time: _____   Blood Sugar:_____
Time: _____   Blood Sugar:_____

Saturday

Time: _____   Blood Sugar:_____
Time: _____   Blood Sugar:_____
Time: _____   Blood Sugar:_____
Time: _____   Blood Sugar:_____

Sunday

Time: _____   Blood Sugar:_____
Time: _____   Blood Sugar:_____
Time: _____   Blood Sugar:_____
Time: _____   Blood Sugar:_____

Notes:

HOME BLOOD SUGAR MONITORING RECORDS

NOVEMBER

▶ Goal values (approximate) <u>**whole blood values:**</u>

1. **Fasting** =100 ± 20 mg/dL. Usually first morning. No food or drink for ≥ 8 hours.
2. **Before meals** = 100 ± 20 mg/dL. Essentially the same as fasting.
3. **Bedtime** = 120 ± 20 mg/dL.
4. **After meal** = 140 mg/dL. Two hours after meals.

▶ Goal values (approximate) <u>**plasma values:**</u>

1. **Fasting** =110 ± 20 mg/dL. Usually first morning. No food or drink for ≥ 8 hours.
2. **Before meals** = 110 ± 20 mg/dL. Essentially the same as fasting.
3. **Bedtime** = 130 ± 20 mg/dL.
4. **After meal** = 150 mg/dL. Two hours after meals.

Monday

Time: _____   Blood Sugar:_____
Time: _____   Blood Sugar:_____
Time: _____   Blood Sugar:_____
Time: _____   Blood Sugar:_____

Tuesday

Time: _____   Blood Sugar:_____
Time: _____   Blood Sugar:_____
Time: _____   Blood Sugar:_____
Time: _____   Blood Sugar:_____

Wednesday

Time: _____   Blood Sugar:_____
Time: _____   Blood Sugar:_____
Time: _____   Blood Sugar:_____
Time: _____   Blood Sugar:_____

Thursday

Time: _____   Blood Sugar:_____
Time: _____   Blood Sugar:_____
Time: _____   Blood Sugar:_____
Time: _____   Blood Sugar:_____

Friday

Time: _____   Blood Sugar:_____
Time: _____   Blood Sugar:_____
Time: _____   Blood Sugar:_____
Time: _____   Blood Sugar:_____

Saturday, November 1:

Time: _____   Blood Sugar:_____
Time: _____   Blood Sugar:_____
Time: _____   Blood Sugar:_____
Time: _____   Blood Sugar:_____

Sunday, November 2:

Time: _____   Blood Sugar:_____
Time: _____   Blood Sugar:_____
Time: _____   Blood Sugar:_____
Time: _____   Blood Sugar:_____

Its time to order your new *DIABETIC DIARY 2004!* 1-877-823-9235

Notes:

Monday, November 3:

Time: _____   Blood Sugar:_____

Time: _____   Blood Sugar:_____

Time: _____   Blood Sugar:_____

Time: _____   Blood Sugar:_____

Tuesday, November 4:

Time: _____   Blood Sugar:_____

Time: _____   Blood Sugar:_____

Time: _____   Blood Sugar:_____

Time: _____   Blood Sugar:_____

Wednesday, November 5:

Time: _____   Blood Sugar:_____

Time: _____   Blood Sugar:_____

Time: _____   Blood Sugar:_____

Time: _____   Blood Sugar:_____

Thursday, November 6:

Time: _____   Blood Sugar:_____

Time: _____   Blood Sugar:_____

Time: _____   Blood Sugar:_____

Time: _____   Blood Sugar:_____

Friday, November 7:

Time: _____   Blood Sugar:_____

Time: _____   Blood Sugar:_____

Time: _____   Blood Sugar:_____

Time: _____   Blood Sugar:_____

Saturday, November 8:

Time: _____   Blood Sugar:_____
Time: _____   Blood Sugar:_____
Time: _____   Blood Sugar:_____
Time: _____   Blood Sugar:_____

Sunday, November 9:

Time: _____   Blood Sugar:_____
Time: _____   Blood Sugar:_____
Time: _____   Blood Sugar:_____
Time: _____   Blood Sugar:_____

Its time to order your new *DIABETIC DIARY 2004!* 1-877-823-9235

Notes:

Monday, November 10:

Time: _____   Blood Sugar:_____
Time: _____   Blood Sugar:_____
Time: _____   Blood Sugar:_____
Time: _____   Blood Sugar:_____

Tuesday, November 11:

Time: _____   Blood Sugar:_____
Time: _____   Blood Sugar:_____
Time: _____   Blood Sugar:_____
Time: _____   Blood Sugar:_____

Wednesday, November 12:

Time: _____   Blood Sugar:_____
Time: _____   Blood Sugar:_____
Time: _____   Blood Sugar:_____
Time: _____   Blood Sugar:_____

Thursday, November 13:

Time: _____   Blood Sugar:_____
Time: _____   Blood Sugar:_____
Time: _____   Blood Sugar:_____
Time: _____   Blood Sugar:_____

Friday, November 14:

Time: _____   Blood Sugar:_____
Time: _____   Blood Sugar:_____
Time: _____   Blood Sugar:_____
Time: _____   Blood Sugar:_____

Saturday, November 15:

Time: _____   Blood Sugar:_____
Time: _____   Blood Sugar:_____
Time: _____   Blood Sugar:_____
Time: _____   Blood Sugar:_____

Sunday, November 16:

Time: _____   Blood Sugar:_____
Time: _____   Blood Sugar:_____
Time: _____   Blood Sugar:_____
Time: _____   Blood Sugar:_____

Its time to order your new *DIABETIC DIARY 2004!* 1-877-823-9235

Notes:

Monday, November 17:

Time: _____ Blood Sugar:_____
Time: _____ Blood Sugar:_____
Time: _____ Blood Sugar:_____
Time: _____ Blood Sugar:_____

Tuesday, November 18:

Time: _____ Blood Sugar:_____
Time: _____ Blood Sugar:_____
Time: _____ Blood Sugar:_____
Time: _____ Blood Sugar:_____

Wednesday, November 19:

Time: _____ Blood Sugar:_____
Time: _____ Blood Sugar:_____
Time: _____ Blood Sugar:_____
Time: _____ Blood Sugar:_____

Thursday, November 20:

Time: _____ Blood Sugar:_____
Time: _____ Blood Sugar:_____
Time: _____ Blood Sugar:_____
Time: _____ Blood Sugar:_____

Friday, November 21:

Time: _____ Blood Sugar:_____
Time: _____ Blood Sugar:_____
Time: _____ Blood Sugar:_____
Time: _____ Blood Sugar:_____

Saturday, November 22:

Time: _____   Blood Sugar:_____
Time: _____   Blood Sugar:_____
Time: _____   Blood Sugar:_____
Time: _____   Blood Sugar:_____

Sunday, November 23:

Time: _____   Blood Sugar:_____
Time: _____   Blood Sugar:_____
Time: _____   Blood Sugar:_____
Time: _____   Blood Sugar:_____

Its time to order your new *DIABETIC DIARY 2004!* 1-877-823-9235

Notes:

Monday, November 24:

Time: _____   Blood Sugar:_____
Time: _____   Blood Sugar:_____
Time: _____   Blood Sugar:_____
Time: _____   Blood Sugar:_____

Tuesday, November 25:

Time: _____   Blood Sugar:_____
Time: _____   Blood Sugar:_____
Time: _____   Blood Sugar:_____
Time: _____   Blood Sugar:_____

Wednesday, November 26:

Time: _____   Blood Sugar:_____
Time: _____   Blood Sugar:_____
Time: _____   Blood Sugar:_____
Time: _____   Blood Sugar:_____

Thursday, November 27:

Time: _____   Blood Sugar:_____
Time: _____   Blood Sugar:_____
Time: _____   Blood Sugar:_____
Time: _____   Blood Sugar:_____

Friday, November 28:

Time: _____   Blood Sugar:_____
Time: _____   Blood Sugar:_____
Time: _____   Blood Sugar:_____
Time: _____   Blood Sugar:_____

Saturday, November 29:

Time: _____   Blood Sugar:_____
Time: _____   Blood Sugar:_____
Time: _____   Blood Sugar:_____
Time: _____   Blood Sugar:_____

Sunday, November 30:

Time: _____   Blood Sugar:_____
Time: _____   Blood Sugar:_____
Time: _____   Blood Sugar:_____
Time: _____   Blood Sugar:_____

Its time to order your new *DIABETIC DIARY 2004!* 1-877-823-9235

Notes:

HOME BLOOD SUGAR MONITORING RECORDS

DECEMBER

▶ Goal values (approximate) <u>**whole blood values:**</u>

1. **Fasting =100 ± 20 mg/dL.** Usually first morning. No food or drink for ≥ 8 hours.

2. **Before meals = 100 ± 20 mg/dL.** Essentially the same as fasting.

3. **Bedtime = 120 ± 20 mg/dL.**

4. **After meal = 140 mg/dL.** Two hours after meals.

▶ Goal values (approximate) <u>**plasma values:**</u>

1. **Fasting =110 ± 20 mg/dL.** Usually first morning. No food or drink for ≥ 8 hours.

2. **Before meals = 110 ± 20 mg/dL.** Essentially the same as fasting.

3. **Bedtime = 130 ± 20 mg/dL.**

4. **After meal = 150 mg/dL.** Two hours after meals.

Monday, December 1:

Time: _____   Blood Sugar:_____
Time: _____   Blood Sugar:_____
Time: _____   Blood Sugar:_____
Time: _____   Blood Sugar:_____

Tuesday, December 2:

Time: _____   Blood Sugar:_____
Time: _____   Blood Sugar:_____
Time: _____   Blood Sugar:_____
Time: _____   Blood Sugar:_____

Wednesday, December 3:

Time: _____   Blood Sugar:_____
Time: _____   Blood Sugar:_____
Time: _____   Blood Sugar:_____
Time: _____   Blood Sugar:_____

Thursday, December 4:

Time: _____   Blood Sugar:_____
Time: _____   Blood Sugar:_____
Time: _____   Blood Sugar:_____
Time: _____   Blood Sugar:_____

Friday, December 5:

Time: _____   Blood Sugar:_____
Time: _____   Blood Sugar:_____
Time: _____   Blood Sugar:_____
Time: _____   Blood Sugar:_____

Saturday, December 6:

Time: _____ Blood Sugar:_____
Time: _____ Blood Sugar:_____
Time: _____ Blood Sugar:_____
Time: _____ Blood Sugar:_____

Sunday, December 7:

Time: _____ Blood Sugar:_____
Time: _____ Blood Sugar:_____
Time: _____ Blood Sugar:_____
Time: _____ Blood Sugar:_____

Its time to order your new *DIABETIC DIARY 2004!* 1-877-823-9235

Notes:

Monday, December 8:

Time: _____ Blood Sugar:_____
Time: _____ Blood Sugar:_____
Time: _____ Blood Sugar:_____
Time: _____ Blood Sugar:_____

Tuesday, December 9:

Time: _____ Blood Sugar:_____
Time: _____ Blood Sugar:_____
Time: _____ Blood Sugar:_____
Time: _____ Blood Sugar:_____

Wednesday, December 10:

Time: _____ Blood Sugar:_____
Time: _____ Blood Sugar:_____
Time: _____ Blood Sugar:_____
Time: _____ Blood Sugar:_____

Thursday, December 11:

Time: _____ Blood Sugar:_____
Time: _____ Blood Sugar:_____
Time: _____ Blood Sugar:_____
Time: _____ Blood Sugar:_____

Friday, December 12:

Time: _____ Blood Sugar:_____
Time: _____ Blood Sugar:_____
Time: _____ Blood Sugar:_____
Time: _____ Blood Sugar:_____

Saturday, December 13:

Time: _____   Blood Sugar:_____
Time: _____   Blood Sugar:_____
Time: _____   Blood Sugar:_____
Time: _____   Blood Sugar:_____

Sunday, December 14:

Time: _____   Blood Sugar:_____
Time: _____   Blood Sugar:_____
Time: _____   Blood Sugar:_____
Time: _____   Blood Sugar:_____

Its time to order your new *DIABETIC DIARY 2004!* 1-877-823-9235

Notes:

Monday, December 15:

Time: _____   Blood Sugar:_____
Time: _____   Blood Sugar:_____
Time: _____   Blood Sugar:_____
Time: _____   Blood Sugar:_____

Tuesday, December 16:

Time: _____   Blood Sugar:_____
Time: _____   Blood Sugar:_____
Time: _____   Blood Sugar:_____
Time: _____   Blood Sugar:_____

Wednesday, December 17:

Time: _____   Blood Sugar:_____
Time: _____   Blood Sugar:_____
Time: _____   Blood Sugar:_____
Time: _____   Blood Sugar:_____

Thursday, December 18:

Time: _____   Blood Sugar:_____
Time: _____   Blood Sugar:_____
Time: _____   Blood Sugar:_____
Time: _____   Blood Sugar:_____

Friday, December 19:

Time: _____   Blood Sugar:_____
Time: _____   Blood Sugar:_____
Time: _____   Blood Sugar:_____
Time: _____   Blood Sugar:_____

Saturday, December 20:
Time: _____ Blood Sugar:_____
Time: _____ Blood Sugar:_____
Time: _____ Blood Sugar:_____
Time: _____ Blood Sugar:_____

Sunday, December 21:
Time: _____ Blood Sugar:_____
Time: _____ Blood Sugar:_____
Time: _____ Blood Sugar:_____
Time: _____ Blood Sugar:_____

Its time to order your new *DIABETIC DIARY 2004!* 1-877-823-9235

Notes:

Monday, December 22:

Time: _____   Blood Sugar:_____
Time: _____   Blood Sugar:_____
Time: _____   Blood Sugar:_____
Time: _____   Blood Sugar:_____

Tuesday, December 23:

Time: _____   Blood Sugar:_____
Time: _____   Blood Sugar:_____
Time: _____   Blood Sugar:_____
Time: _____   Blood Sugar:_____

Wednesday, December 24:

Time: _____   Blood Sugar:_____
Time: _____   Blood Sugar:_____
Time: _____   Blood Sugar:_____
Time: _____   Blood Sugar:_____

Thursday, December 25:

Time: _____   Blood Sugar:_____
Time: _____   Blood Sugar:_____
Time: _____   Blood Sugar:_____
Time: _____   Blood Sugar:_____

Friday, December 26:

Time: _____   Blood Sugar:_____
Time: _____   Blood Sugar:_____
Time: _____   Blood Sugar:_____
Time: _____   Blood Sugar:_____

Saturday, December 27:

Time: _____   Blood Sugar:_____
Time: _____   Blood Sugar:_____
Time: _____   Blood Sugar:_____
Time: _____   Blood Sugar:_____

Sunday, December 28:

Time: _____   Blood Sugar:_____
Time: _____   Blood Sugar:_____
Time: _____   Blood Sugar:_____
Time: _____   Blood Sugar:_____

Its time to order your new *DIABETIC DIARY 2004!* 1-877-823-9235

Notes:

Monday, December29:

Time: _____   Blood Sugar:_____
Time: _____   Blood Sugar:_____
Time: _____   Blood Sugar:_____
Time: _____   Blood Sugar:_____

Tuesday, December 30:

Time: _____   Blood Sugar:_____
Time: _____   Blood Sugar:_____
Time: _____   Blood Sugar:_____
Time: _____   Blood Sugar:_____

Wednesday, December 31:

Time: _____   Blood Sugar:_____
Time: _____   Blood Sugar:_____
Time: _____   Blood Sugar:_____
Time: _____   Blood Sugar:_____

Thursday

Time: _____   Blood Sugar:_____
Time: _____   Blood Sugar:_____
Time: _____   Blood Sugar:_____
Time: _____   Blood Sugar:_____

Friday

Time: _____   Blood Sugar:_____
Time: _____   Blood Sugar:_____
Time: _____   Blood Sugar:_____
Time: _____   Blood Sugar:_____

Saturday:

Time: _____   Blood Sugar:_____
Time: _____   Blood Sugar:_____
Time: _____   Blood Sugar:_____
Time: _____   Blood Sugar:_____

Sunday:

Time: _____   Blood Sugar:_____
Time: _____   Blood Sugar:_____
Time: _____   Blood Sugar:_____
Time: _____   Blood Sugar:_____

Its time to order your new *DIABETIC DIARY 2004!* 1-877-823-9235

Notes:

WEIGHTS

▶ Checks for risk of worsening diabetes.

▶ Recording your weights monthly should be adequate.

▶ Weight management is important, especially in Type 2 diabetes. Obese Type 2 diabetics can significantly improve their blood sugar control and even cure their diabetes with weight reduction. Conversely, weight gain can contribute to uncontrolled diabetes and subsequent complications.

▶ Calculate your body mass index (BMI) from the following formula:

BMI = weight _____ Kg ÷ (height _____ meters)^2

Normal is BMI ≤ 25.

Overweight is BMI between 25 and 30.

Obese is BMI ≥ 30.

▶ Conversion from English units is easy.

Weight _____ lb. ÷ 2.2 = _____ Kg.

Height _____ in. x 2.54 ÷ 100 = _____ meters.

WEIGHTS

January:

_____ lb.
_____ Kg.
_____ BMI

February:

_____ lb.
_____ Kg.
_____ BMI

March:

_____ lb.
_____ Kg.
_____ BMI

April:

_____ lb.
_____ Kg.
_____ BMI

May:

_____ lb.
_____ Kg.
_____ BMI

June:

_____ lb.
_____ Kg.
_____ BMI

July:

_____ lb.
_____ Kg.
_____ BMI

August:

_____ lb.
_____ Kg.
_____ BMI

September:

_____ lb.
_____ Kg.
_____ BMI

October:

_____ lb.
_____ Kg.
_____ BMI

November:

_____ lb.
_____ Kg.
_____ BMI

December:

_____ lb.
_____ Kg.
_____ BMI

BLOOD PRESSURE

▶ Checks risk for heart disease, stroke and kidney disease.

▶ Record your blood pressures as measured by a health care professional monthly should be adequate. Your physician may monitor your blood pressure more frequently until it is under control. You may use an average if your health care provider measures several readings during one visit.

▶ Current recommendations:
Systolic Blood Pressure ≤ 130 (top number).
Diastolic Blood Pressure ≤ 80 (bottom number).

BLOOD PRESSURE

January:

_____ mm Hg Systolic
_____ mm Hg Diastolic

February:

_____ mm Hg Systolic
_____ mm Hg Diastolic

March:

_____ mm Hg Systolic
_____ mm Hg Diastolic

April:

_____ mm Hg Systolic
_____ mm Hg Diastolic

May:

_____ mm Hg Systolic
_____ mm Hg Diastolic

June:

_____ mm Hg Systolic
_____ mm Hg Diastolic

July:

_____ mm Hg Systolic
_____ mm Hg Diastolic

August:

_____ mm Hg Systolic
_____ mm Hg Diastolic

September:

_____ mm Hg Systolic
_____ mm Hg Diastolic

October:

_____ mm Hg Systolic
_____ mm Hg Diastolic

November:

_____ mm Hg Systolic
_____ mm Hg Diastolic

December:

_____ mm Hg Systolic
_____ mm Hg Diastolic

HEMOGLOBIN A$_1$C
(GLYCOSYLATED HEMOGLOBIN)

▶ Measures average blood sugar control over the preceding 2 or 3 months.

▶ Record values in the corresponding month in which they were tested.

▶ Measurement is recommended twice yearly if sugar control is stable and quarterly if treatment goals aren't met or if therapy is changed.

▶ **As a general rule, therapeutic blood sugar control is indicated by a result of ≤ 7%. Change in therapy is indicated at values ≥ 8%.**

▶ Note: There is a lack of standardization between assays, so your doctor may make recommendations idiosyncratic to the assay used.

HEMOGLOBIN A$_1$C
(GLYCOSYLATED HEMOGLOBIN)

January:................._____ %

February:............._____ %

March: ...._____ %

April: ...._____ %

May: ...._____ %

June: ...._____ %

July: ...._____ %

August: ...._____ %

September: ...._____ %

October: ...._____ %

November: ...._____ %

December: ...._____ %

LIPIDS

▶ Checks risk for heart disease and stroke.

▶ Record values in the corresponding month in which they were tested.

▶ Generally, adult diabetic patients should have their lipids checked yearly. Lipids that should be measured include LDL-cholesterol (bad cholesterol), HDL-cholesterol (good cholesterol) and triglycerides. Children > 2 year of age may be screened.

▶ If the resultant values fall into the low risk category (LDL-C < 100 mg/dL, HDL-C > 45 mg/dL for men and > 55 mg/dL for women, triglycerides <200) screening can be performed every 2 years.

▶ Testing may be indicated more often when being pharmacologically treated for high risk lipid levels, especially in the initiation stages.

▶ Therapeutic goals include
LDL-cholesterol < 100 mg/dL
HDL-cholesterol > 45 mg/dL for men and >55 mg/dL for women
Triglycerides < 200 mg/dL

▶ If treated pharmacologically other tests may be indicated, most commonly the transaminases ALT (alanine aminotransferase) and AST (aspartame aminotransferase) to monitor liver function and CK (creatine kinase) to monitor skeletal muscle biochemistry. Space is included for these test results.

LIPIDS

January:

LDL-C ...._____ mg/dl   ALT ...._____ IU/dl
HDL-C...._____ mg/dl   AST ...._____ IU/dl
Trig. ...._____ mg/dl   CK......_____ IU/dl

February:

LDL-C ...._____ mg/dl   ALT ...._____ IU/dl
HDL-C...._____ mg/dl   AST ...._____ IU/dl
Trig. ...._____ mg/dl   CK......_____ IU/dl

March:

LDL-C ...._____ mg/dl   ALT ...._____ IU/dl
HDL-C...._____ mg/dl   AST ...._____ IU/dl
Trig. ...._____ mg/dl   CK......_____ IU/dl

April:

LDL-C ...._____ mg/dl   ALT ...._____ IU/dl
HDL-C...._____ mg/dl   AST ...._____ IU/dl
Trig. ...._____ mg/dl   CK......_____ IU/dl

May:

LDL-C ...._____ mg/dl   ALT ...._____ IU/dl
HDL-C...._____ mg/dl   AST ...._____ IU/dl
Trig. ...._____ mg/dl   CK......_____ IU/dl

June:

LDL-C ...._____ mg/dl   ALT ...._____ IU/dl
HDL-C...._____ mg/dl   AST ...._____ IU/dl
Trig. ...._____ mg/dl   CK......_____ IU/dl

LIPIDS

July:

LDL-C ...._____ mg/dl   ALT ...._____ IU/dl
HDL-C...._____ mg/dl   AST ...._____ IU/dl
Trig. ...._____ mg/dl   CK......_____ IU/dl

August:

LDL-C ...._____ mg/dl   ALT ...._____ IU/dl
HDL-C...._____ mg/dl   AST ...._____ IU/dl
Trig. ...._____ mg/dl   CK......_____ IU/dl

September:

LDL-C ...._____ mg/dl   ALT ...._____ IU/dl
HDL-C...._____ mg/dl   AST ...._____ IU/dl
Trig. ...._____ mg/dl   CK......_____ IU/dl

October:

LDL-C ...._____ mg/dl   ALT ...._____ IU/dl
HDL-C...._____ mg/dl   AST ...._____ IU/dl
Trig. ...._____ mg/dl   CK......_____ IU/dl

November:

LDL-C ...._____ mg/dl   ALT ...._____ IU/dl
HDL-C...._____ mg/dl   AST ...._____ IU/dl
Trig. ...._____ mg/dl   CK......_____ IU/dl

December:

LDL-C ...._____ mg/dl   ALT ...._____ IU/dl
HDL-C...._____ mg/dl   AST ...._____ IU/dl
Trig. ...._____ mg/dl   CK......_____ IU/dl

Urinary Microalbumin

_____Check here if your doctor has diagnosed you with gross proteinuria and skip this section

▶ Checks kidney (renal function)

▶ Record values in the corresponding month in which they were tested.

▶ Urinalysis should be performed yearly. If no protein is detected then a follow up test should be performed looking for small amounts of albumin, called microalbumin. The test can be performed in any of three ways.

1. Random first morning urine sample is the most common and convenient method used. If a first morning specimen is not possible, urine samples should be obtained at the same time of day for meaningful comparisons. The creatinine in the urine is also measured and the result is reported as a ratio.
   Normal value is < 30 μg/mg.

2. Twenty four hour collection. Urine is collected for 24 hours and analyzed for the total albumin.
   Normal value is <30 mg/24 hr.

3. Timed collection over 4 or 8 hours.
   Normal value is <20 μg/min.

▶ Because of normal variability, 2 of 3 specimens over a 3 to 6 month period should be abnormal before this test is considered positive. Exercise, infection, fever, congestive heart failure, severe hyperglycemia and severe hypertension can cause false positives.

URINARY MICROALBUMIN

January:

_____ µg/mg
_____ mg/hr
_____ µg/min

February:

_____ µg/mg
_____ mg/hr
_____ µg/min

March:

_____ µg/mg
_____ mg/hr
_____ µg/min

April:

_____ µg/mg
_____ mg/hr
_____ µg/min

May:

_____ µg/mg
_____ mg/hr
_____ µg/min

June:

_____ µg/mg
_____ mg/hr
_____ µg/min

July:

_____ µg/mg
_____ mg/hr
_____ µg/min

August:

_____ µg/mg
_____ mg/hr
_____ µg/min

September:

_____ µg/mg
_____ mg/hr
_____ µg/min

October:

_____ µg/mg
_____ mg/hr
_____ µg/min

November:

_____ µg/mg
_____ mg/hr
_____ µg/min

December:

_____ µg/mg
_____ mg/hr
_____ µg/min

Kidney (Renal) Function

▶ Record values in the corresponding month in which they were tested.

▶ There are no specific recommendations for testing intervals, but your physician should be checking these values, especially if you are on certain medications such as metformin (Glucophage) and ACE inhibitors.

▶ Another measurement of kidney function is blood urea nitrogen (BUN) and creatinine (CRT). Especially if you are taking a blood pressure medication called ACE inhibitors (angiotensin converting enzyme inhibitors) you should have your BUN, CRT and K (potassium) checked 2-3 weeks after initiation of the medication and 2-3 weeks after any dose change, then periodically.

KIDNEY (RENAL) FUNCTION

January:

_____ mg/dl
_____ mg/dl
_____ meq/dl

February:

_____ mg/dl
_____ mg/dl
_____ meq/dl

March:

_____ mg/dl
_____ mg/dl
_____ meq/dl

April:

_____ mg/dl
_____ mg/dl
_____ meq/dl

May:

_____ mg/dl
_____ mg/dl
_____ meq/dl

June:

_____ mg/dl
_____ mg/dl
_____ meq/dl

July:

_____ mg/dl
_____ mg/dl
_____ meq/dl

August:

_____ mg/dl
_____ mg/dl
_____ meq/dl

September:

_____ mg/dl
_____ mg/dl
_____ meq/dl

October:

_____ mg/dl
_____ mg/dl
_____ meq/dl

November:

_____ mg/dl
_____ mg/dl
_____ meq/dl

December:

_____ mg/dl
_____ mg/dl
_____ meq/dl

EXAMINATIONS

▶ Record your physicians names in the space provided.

▶ Check the month(s) corresponding to examination dates.

▶ **General diabetic examinations:**

1. **Twice yearly** if your diabetes is controlled.

2. **Quarterly** if not meeting therapeutic goals. More often if prescribed.

▶ **Diabetic foot examinations:**

1. **Your feet should be examined at every doctor visit!** It is best just to get into the habit of taking your shoes and socks off every time you see your doctor!

2. **A yearly examination** by a foot specialist such as a *podiatrist, orthopedic surgeon or vascular surgeon* is recommended by some.

▶ **Diabetic eye examinations:**

1. **Yearly** by an *ophthalmologist*; more often if prescribed. Diabetes is still the most common cause of blindness world wide.

GENERAL DIABETIC EXAMINATIONS

January: _____

February: _____

March: _____

April: _____

May: _____

June: _____

July: _____

August: _____

September: _____

October: _____

November: _____

December: _____

Diabetes physician _____

DIABETIC FOOT EXAMINATIONS

January: _____

February: _____

March: _____

April: _____

May: _____

June: _____

July: _____

August: _____

September: _____

October: _____

November: _____

December: _____

Diabetes foot specialist _____

DIABETIC EYE EXAMINATIONS

January: _____

February: _____

March: _____

April: _____

May: _____

June: _____

July: _____

August: _____

September: _____

October: _____

November: _____

December: _____

Ophthalmologist_____

REFERENCES

1. American Diabetic Association. www.diabetes.org. August 2003 review of Position statements, Consensus statements and Technical reviews.

2. American Diabetic Association. www.diabetes.org. August 2002 review of Position statements, Consensus statements and Technical reviews.

3. American Diabetic Association. www.diabetes.org. August 2001 review of Position statements, Consensus statements and Technical reviews.

4. ABCNEWS.com. Fending off the Flu, New Pill Works Like Vaccine, 20 November 2000.

5. American Family Physician. Alternative Therapies: Part I. Depression, Diabetes, Obesity. 1 September 2000.

6. American Family Physician. Diagnosis and Classification of Diabetes Mellitus New Criteria. 15 October 1998

7. American Family Physician. New Oral Therapies for Type 2 Diabetes. 1 November 1997.

7. American Family Physician. New Treatments for Diabetes. 15 May 1999.

9. American Family Physician. Oral Pharmacological of Type 2 Diabetes. 1 December 1999.

10. American Family Physician. Use of ACE Inhibitors in Patients with Type 2 Diabetes. 1 May 2000.

About the Author

L. D. Sutton, M.D., Ph.D.

Dr. Sutton is a physician-scientist with 58 scientific publications and presentations to his credit. He received his Medical Degree from the University of Iowa College of Medicine and his Doctoral of Philosophy degree from the University of Iowa College of Liberal Arts' Department of Chemistry. He completed specialty training in Clinical Pathology at the University of Iowa Hospitals and Clinics and in Family Practice at Broadlawns Medical Center in Des Moines, Iowa. His practice experience includes faculty positions in pathology at both the University of Arkansas for Medical Sciences and the University of Iowa Hospitals and Clinics, Director of Clinical Microbiology at the McClellan Memorial Veteran's Administration Hospital in Little Rock, Arkansas and a successful private practice in Family and Emergency Medicine. After serving as Senior Research Scientist for Bio-Research Products, Inc., he co-founded Joel Health Industries, Inc. where he currently works as President.